VOYAGE TO THE ISLAND

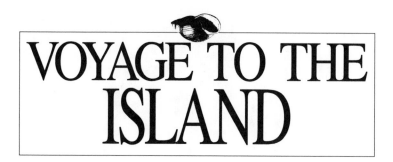

VOYAGE TO THE ISLAND

Raija Nieminen

Translated by Raili Ojala
with assistance from
Carolyn B. Norris

Gallaudet University Press
Washington, D.C.

Gallaudet University Press, Washington, DC 20002
© 1990 by Gallaudet University. All rights reserved
Published 1990
Printed in the United States of America
Originally published 1985 by Tammi Publishers, Helsinki, Finland

Library of Congress Cataloging-in-Publication Data

Nieminen, Raija.
   [Äänetön saari]
   Voyage to the island / Raija Nieminen ; translated by Raili Ojala,
with assistance from Carolyn B. Norris.
   p.   cm.
   Translation of: Äänetön saari.
   ISBN 0-930323-62-9
   1. Nieminen, Raija. 2. Deaf—Finland—Biography. 3. Deaf—Saint
Lucia. 4. Deaf—Education—Saint Lucia.   I. Title.
HV2785.5.N54   1990
362.4′2′092—dc20
   [B]   90-19178
                                                     CIP

Photographs by Johanna Mesch, Clyde Vincent, and Jukka Nieminen.

VOYAGE TO THE
ISLAND

TO ST. LUCIA

Study abroad – what will you be leaving behind?

I am floating in a huge British Airways jet above clouds and sea; stewardesses are busy in the aisle. I feel calm. I have left behind the old familiar world and am on my way to something completely different. The dark-complexioned, colorfully dressed passengers around me, the strange fragrances of their perfumes and soaps, their gestures and facial expressions belong to the place I'm heading toward.

It's all the same to me what language is being spoken around me. The stewardess may ask in any language if I want coffee or tea. I turn my head and look at my sons, Keke, 16, and Joppe, 13. One or the other of them repeats the question to me. They never need to speak especially slowly or clearly because I've watched their lips for years, and I know how they form the unheard sounds.

The passengers listen to music to pass the time, hearing through the earphones that the steward in first class has distributed to them. I am the only one without earphones. Once in a while I still long for music, and often the humming in my ears changes into music, playing pieces that I heard a long time ago, when my auditory nerves still could sense sound vibrations. Keke is tapping absentmindedly on the arm of his seat, and I feel with him the rhythm of the music.

otic scticl We are flying toward the sun and toward a strange country, the tropical island of St. Lucia, of which we know only the name. I am waiting for the moment when the island will appear suddenly below us, in the middle of the shining sea, from beneath the purple evening clouds, a breathtaking sight of yellow beaches and swaying palms.

My watch still shows the time of the old world. We've been on the way for fifteen hours, including a stop in London. It should be night now, but it's still afternoon. This November day in 1975 is the longest day in my life so far. But it has seemed short.

After the English afternoon tea, the plane turns to the right. The island appears as expected, a tiny piece of land sitting hunched in the dusk under the rainclouds; on the left, two huge mountains rise, all out of proportion. How can the huge plane land on such a small piece of land? But soon we are whizzing along the runway. Our island looks deserted and mysterious and not beautiful at all.

Suddenly it's almost dark. The lights of the runway are turned on, and the asphalt shines after the rain. I put on my cardigan, and we collect our belongings and step onto the soil of the new country. The air is wet and warm. The invigorating freezing weather we're used to belongs to the world that we left behind, where the night now is already deep, far away beyond the blue sea and the clouds.

Jukka, my husband, is standing on the terrace of the airport, waving. He has come two weeks earlier to start a development project on the island, to improve the port. I shake my head to the stewardess who is giving out transit cards at the gate. No, we are not continuing our journey. We will stay here for at least two years. There are many islands in the Caribbean, and the plane will land on several more of them on its way to British Guyana. We will stay here in this *fear, anticipation* hot, wet country with lizards, millipedes, poisonous spiders, and snakes. It is our new world. I am well prepared for it; everything we will need is in my bags: medicine, insecticide, disinfectants. When I thought beforehand of our new life, I was sometimes afraid. But now that I'm here, everything seems much simpler. Of course we'll survive.

The customs officer thinks I'm too well prepared. Fortunately Jukka pushes through to the customs counter and explains that we will indeed need this and that in the next two years. The customs officer doesn't know yet that the two wooden boxes being ferried from the plane also contain our things. Keke is worrying about his guitar because its bag lost all its labels warning about fragility.

The small St. Lucia Airways plane at the side of the runway seems like a hummingbird next to the huge sea-eagle on which we have travelled this far. It makes me a little nervous when the hummingbird buzzes along the runway and rises, swaying, above the palms. In the darkness below us the sea glimmers. The plane is a frail bird above the silhouettes of the dark island and its mountains and palms.

I try to see what Jukka is saying.

"We're flying around the island—it's safer than flying directly over the mountains."

I am already so used to seeing what Jukka says that the light from the small lamp above the door leading to the cockpit is enough. I don't need to say, "It's too dark for me to hear."

Jukka presses my hand for me to look at his face. "We'll soon fly over the town of Castries. Look for the lights; they'll be visible soon, down in the valley."

I hold my breath. Light belts twist and turn from the valley to the surrounding mountains. It reminds me of the trip on Jukka's boat through the Strait of Messina: the towns on each side of the strait were light masses climbing up the mountain.

The runway of the small airport near Castries starts straight from the sea. On the sides of the runway the trees are flickering before my eyes—beyond the trees there's only darkness.

We walk through a noisy group of men. I wonder what they want from me? A man in a white uniform and a big black helmet appears with a whip in his hand and tries to keep order. Jukka arrives with the bags and explains that the men are taxi drivers who are fighting over customers. But Jukka has his car; we don't need a taxi.

The cars passing us on the other side of the road seem to be driving straight toward us because we're driving on the left side of the road. I wonder what this island is like, what is life like inside its houses? Everything is covered by the soft, wet darkness. In the beams of the headlights I can only see fluttering insects. The branches bending over the road are full of big tropical flowers. Where is Jukka taking us, his wife and two sons? I hope he has at least found us a decent home.

Jukka stops the car. On the slope beneath us there is a white house we can reach by climbing down some steps. A part of the house is hanging on the slope, resting on tall, thin pillars. I step down carefully, so curious that I forget to take my share of the bags. Jukka left the porch light on, so we can see. There are shells, snails, and worms on the stairs, and black caterpillars with countless feet on the walls. But the spiders that I dread are nowhere in sight.

I examine the whole house bit by bit and am happily surprised. Everything is clean and tidy: three rooms plus a kitchen and a bathroom. There is a gas stove and a refrigerator in the kitchen, hot water and a shower in the bathroom. The windows have glass trellises, called espaliers. The cottage is owned by an American couple, the Rogerses, who spend two months on the island every winter.

One wall in the living room is made of bricks with large holes in them. All kinds of creeping things can come in through the holes. Mosquitoes are already flying around the room. I dig out the mosquito repellent from my bag, and everyone spreads it on. There are hooks above the beds to tie the mosquito nets to, later on when we go to bed.

"There are red bees here. You have to look out for them," Jukka says. And later, "Our house has its own good guardian, a green lizard. It stops by once in a while to greet us."

At night I wake up, feeling hungry. My stomach is still on the old-world time, and at this hour in the old world I would be sitting at the kitchen table having my breakfast, reading my newspaper. I spread more mosquito repellent on and walk carefully, with my eyes on the floor the whole time. Before this trip I read in a guidebook that one should never walk barefoot on the floor. Keke is sitting in the kitchen, reading and munching cookies. His stomach has also reminded him of the time difference.

I wake up again at seven o'clock; it's light, but the light from the sun that dwells behind the mountain is pale and hasn't yet warmed up. Below the shore under the palms people are taking their morning swim.

observation Jukka prepares breakfast. He is mixing milk from powder; he pours boiled water into drinking bottles to cool.

"Remember that ice cubes also have to be made of boiled water. Teeth can be brushed with unboiled water, if it isn't too brown."

Cornflakes, boiled eggs, coffee, and toast. The kitchen is still clean and unoccupied. Dishes are stacked in neat piles, and there are unopened boxes of cookies and cornflakes in the clean cupboards. A big green grasshopper sits motionless on the ceiling; a colorless frog jumps in between the espalier and the window.

deafness helps her adjust to some deafness)

"There was a horrible noise last night, I couldn't sleep at all," Jukka said. The boys were complaining about the same thing; I know what they're thinking. Lucky me who can sleep in peace without being disturbed by the night sounds of the tropics.

Jukka goes to work a little before eight, leaving us to get used to everything that's different: a new house, strange trees, unusual flowers and birds, warm sun, strong smells.

I take a cup of coffee and go to the balcony. The sun has come out from behind the mountains. The sea is shining turquoise, the palms are waving on the golden beach. In the valley lies the town of Castries, which I saw yesterday only as a mass of lights. The sun is shining even hotter now, but then a refreshing wind begins to blow.

The red bees start to buzz; The green lizard climbs along the porch rail and stares with its black eyes. Suddenly it gets frightened and swells its neck into a yellow balloon. Beautiful small animal, I like it right away. I already like this whole place.

Yet, later on in the day, I am overtaken by longing. What have we begun! Two years in this strange country, in the midst of strange things, so far from Finland!

can't hear) - actually makes adjustment easier

mixed reactions)

1st reac — delight, pleasure

WONDERS OF THE ISLAND

initial enchantment

Soon we'll get to know the wonders of the island: the rain that comes from the mountains like a gray wall, sometimes stopping a few meters before it reaches our house, sometimes falling on the roof in a heavy downpour. The clouds hang between the cone-shaped mountains, and the sun shines almost all the time over nearby Pigeon Island. A huge, complete rainbow stretches from the dimly visible neighboring island all the way to Gros Piton and Petit Piton in the distance.

The rain forests seem to whirl down the sides of the mountains. Alamandas and hibiscus glow at the hotel swimming pools, large and small birds quiver among the flowers. In the evening, in the dark, the fireflies flash their lanterns. A huge moon sometimes rises from behind the mountains. The palms shimmer in its light, and the sky is completely full of stars; at the skyline, the black mountain silhouettes rise from the horizon.

The roads wind up to the mountains. We dash up and down again; I hold on to my seat and my breath catches. When the car slows down I can see the scenery below: turquoise sea-bays, the white town, boats in the harbor, and sailboats at anchor; in the deep blue-green of the valleys, the starlike tops of the palms and banana trees form a natural geometry.

People on the island are as colorful as the Nature around them. The women wear bright cotton dresses; they are slim, and beautiful-limbed, with elastic steps. They walk erect and proud, carrying baskets or water dishes on their heads.

The peace of Sunday morning resembles that of my childhood, when I was dressed in a clean summer dress and taken to church. The island people walk along the sunny road in their Sunday dresses, on their way to church with their used black Bibles and songbooks in their hands.

There's so much beauty, and although we get used to it all, the first impressions still remain as wonders.

St. Lucia (pronounced Saint Loosha) is an island about 60 kilometers long and 20 kilometers wide. It is one of the Windward Islands, part of the Lesser Antilles, which are lined up like a string of pearls to the south of the large islands of the West Indies: Cuba, Haiti, and Jamaica. St. Lucia is formed out of a group of volcanic mountains rising from the sea. Because of the mountains it rains a lot in St. Lucia, and the vegetation is exuberant.

The tropical climate makes life different from what we were used to in Finland. We have to learn how to live on the island. The drinking water has to be boiled and milk made out of powder. Clothes and shoes have to be checked once in a while and kept as dry as possible so they won't get moldy. The air is wet all the time, especially during the rainy season. A slight smell of mold mixes with the smell of tropical flowers and trees. The temperature is about 80 degrees, the sun is so hot that the rocks burn our hands. We must avoid getting too much sun and remember to drink enough. A soft wind that cools down the heat is always blowing from the northeast.

Jukka began his work in the Port Office right after he arrived. In the bay, Nature has formed a deep, safe, and sheltered harbor that pushes itself into the middle of the town. The harbor basin is an old volcanic crater. The sea and the port are essential to life on the island. Exports and imports come and go by sea, and most of the tourists, who are important to the economy of the island, arrive on Caribbean cruise ships.

New piers and warehouses are being built in the harbor. The Port Authority asked the United Nations for an expert to look after the enlargement of the port, to plan the administration, and to train the personnel. Jukka applied for the job, and as a result of a long selection process, we are now here.

"Such a young man we got. We expected to get a bit older one," said the director of a local stevedoring company when Jukka arrived. But I know what will happen; they will see what this young man is like!

Jukka is not just an advisor on the island, he is the general manager of the Port Authority, a government office under the Ministry of Communication,

Works, and Labor. He will need to get acquainted with the situation in the port, familiarize himself with matters, interview people, and take notes.

"Everybody says that here in the warm climate one has to work in a lower gear," he says.

Keke and Joppe also have to start working—to study English. Joppe was only in the seventh grade when we left Finland and doesn't even know all the tenses of English verbs. Keke had started high school, so he has a better grounding in English. In St. Lucia they follow the British educational system, in which there are three three-month terms in the year and a month's vacation between them. Christmas vacation will start soon, so there's no use in the boys going to school yet. Instead they will have a governess. Mrs. Glace comes every morning at ten. She plays games with the boys and tries to get them to argue with her. Mrs. Glace seems to have found the right way to get the boys to converse in English.

For my part, I learn to be lazy, because according to local custom, we have a maid. Zenia comes every morning, at eight o'clock at first, then at eight-thirty, then later, according to another local custom. Nobody seems to be in a hurry, yet all occasions start on this timetable, and people arrive appropriately. When you get used to it, it feels good.

On sunny mornings I watch Zenia walk up the hill, slowly, saving her energy. It's the way the islanders have of walking up the slopes of the high mountains. Zenia is carrying a brown paper bag in her hand. She has bought mangoes, bananas, avocados, and many other kinds of fruit that I've never seen before.

One afternoon, Keke buys a big bunch of green "bananas" surprisingly cheap. We wait for them to ripen and become juicy and sweet. But they don't ripen or turn yellow, because we find out, they're not bananas, but plantains. Zenia is also our cook; she prepares the plantains in salt water or fries them crisp in coconut oil. She makes thick yellow soup out of big pumpkin slices.

One day I see Zenia leaning on the stair rail, talking to a dark-skinned man, much darker than she.

Joppe interprets when the man starts talking to me.

"My name is Anderson," he laughs; his teeth are shining white.

Joppe explains that Anderson is a gardener, and that he takes care of many gardens in this part of the town. It was Anderson who mentioned this house to

Jukka when he was driving around here searching for a place for us. Besides that, it was Anderson who arranged for Zenia to work for us.

After that, when we walk down the hill to go swimming at Vigie Beach, the boys tug my hand at the curve in the road. I turn my head and see Anderson's laughing face from behind the hedge. I guess what Anderson is saying: "Good afternoon, Madame."

When it's raining Zenia doesn't come to work at all, because when it rains over here it pours down rain. It's November and the rainy season has started. The whole town is flooding. Soil is rolling down from the mountain slopes, and roads are blocked. The boys from the nearby St. Mary's College usually walk up our hill to school in the mornings, but some mornings there's nobody to be seen. On the worst rainy days, the government orders the schools to be closed. The school closing is announced on the radio in the mornings. All important announcements here are read on the radio.

We sit inside when the rain is pouring down. We don't have anything to do. The air is dripping moisture, even in the house.

In the evenings, we often think of Jeri, our big, black Rottweiler. He is in Finland with Jukka's sister Leena and her family, who are living at our house and looking after everything while we're gone. We miss our loyal friend Jeri, whose lively nature brought coziness and safety to our house. 🐾

BETWEEN TWO WORLDS

[handwritten: probs of speechreading diff language]

St. Lucia has been a British colony for over a century, and its official language is English. I understand written English, but I can't read this language from the lips at all. I have a feeling that I never will learn. English sounds look so different from the familiar Finnish sounds that I can see on the lips if they are pronounced even a little clearly. But here the *o* is different from the *o* in our language; all the vowels are different. The consonants in English can't be seen from behind the teeth at all, except *th*, which seems to slip in between the teeth, but too fast.

[handwritten margin: new lang + new probs on speechread]

That's why I don't understand Zenia's speech at all in the beginning. Little by little I understand a word here and there, but it's not enough.

Speaking English is also difficult. I have to watch where the tongue is and how the lips are, but it isn't enough. I pronounce the language the best I know how, and to my great surprise Zenia understands almost everything I tell her. Sometimes I tell her long stories from my home country. Here it's like this and like that, but everything is completely different in Finland, and I have to tell this to someone. So far Zenia is the only one I can talk to. She washes dishes in the kitchen, sweeps the stairs and cement corridors, washes clothes—I can always find her.

[handwritten margin: Zenia accepts]

Only 2 percent of the inhabitants of the island are white. They all know each other, and soon they'll know that a new family has arrived.

One day Jukka tells me during his lunch hour that a woman (I can't read names from the lips and sometimes I suggest to Jukka that he could learn to fingerspell names for me) sent another woman to ask Jukka whether they could help me in any way.

[handwritten: deaf ignorance about deafness?]

can tell what [a] person's legal attitude is — prob. w/ deaf or simple

How friendly, but . . .

Of course a new inhabitant needs information about this or that. People in other parts of the world are polite and want to help new neighbors in a way I'm not used to in Finland. Perhaps I need to find out where I can find a cookbook, or mutton, or where to find the library, or a hairdresser, or a dentist.

friendliness deaf

But this Mrs. Somebody might also imagine that I live somewhere inside walls where I have to wait until somebody comes and takes me by the hand and helps me do everything. I don't hear, you know. But, I am able to take care of everything myself. I go to town and buy food, sheets, and dishes. We don't need much because the house is completely furnished. I sleep, wake up, eat, arrange the rooms, take care of business. In my opinion I live just like everybody else.

The best way you can help me is by speaking clearly when you meet me. You can face me when you speak so that I see your face the whole time, and you can form letters clearly on your lips so that they can be distinguished from each other. Perhaps you might take a pen and paper from your bag and write what you want to say. It would help me if you could learn which are my difficulties and which are not.

clear advice

But first we have to make this clear to all the people we meet.

We meet Mrs. X and Mr. Y and Miss Z. English, American, Canadian; locals. They are polite, smiling people who ask me something after the introduction. I'm usually asked first how I like it on St. Lucia. I don't need to say anything but "Very well, thank you."

people's misund- husb. must explain

But I don't say anything in the beginning; I just let Jukka do the interpreting.

I look at Jukka, and Jukka says, "Mrs. X is asking how you like it on the island."

"Very much, thank you," I answer.

"Your wife doesn't speak English?"

Jukka smiles and begins, "My wife . . ." Patiently Jukka repeats his story about me, over and over again. He tries his best to explain how normal and usual I am, and in Jukka's opinion even slightly more normal than average. I know English and German, Swedish and sign language, Finnish and soon, perhaps, even American with its fingerspelling and American signs. But to be able to understand conversation, I have to learn to lipread English. And then the climax:

get people to accept . . .

I can read Finnish from the lips even from twenty meters away! Jukka repeats his old story about the time we were sitting in a restaurant and I told him what the couple on the other side of the room was talking about.

At this point everybody is so surprised that some of their prejudices have been forgotten. They are wondering at the simple fact that English is not our first language.

Again and again I wonder about Jukka. He is able to look at the world as if from a watchtower, seeing people and things in their proper proportions. His starting point always is what I am able to do and what possibilities I have, not just the fact that I don't hear. If all hearing people could have this kind of attitude, there wouldn't be such a huge gap between deaf and hearing people. And I wouldn't need to hang in between the two worlds as I do now.

Sometimes I get tired of always being on a journey, going back and forth between the deaf and hearing worlds because I can't completely belong to either of them. Transition is sometimes difficult. I have come home from visiting my friends, from a committee meeting of the Deaf Association, from the celebration at the Deaf Club, or from a class. My friends have talked with their hands and hearts and with their whole person. I feel warm and light.

I remember, back in Finland, Jeri would meet me at the door, jumping up on me eagerly. Jukka and the boys would be happy to see me. It's as warm and safe at home for me as it is in the deaf world in Finland. I don't feel disabled. But when I have to go out and run some errands or go to my part-time job, it doesn't take long for the coldness of the other, hearing world to hit me. People there usually speak with "too small a mouth," as we put it. The world has been made so that most things are based on hearing, not on seeing, although it just as well could be the opposite.

Now, here on the island, I'm once again in a completely new situation. Here everything is different, and I don't know yet whether it will be easier or more difficult. My whole life has been built out of small worlds, each of which I have gotten used to separately. I have to travel between them, and that has required a lot of my energy.

When I was young I thought that everything was as it should have been, but once in a while I had a feeling that I was alone and had walls around me— although I tried to behave as if they didn't exist. I didn't understand how many sounds there were in the world that I didn't hear. Over time, the wall grew even bigger and closed more and more sounds out of my hearing, although I didn't quite understand what it was all about.

My auditory nerves deteriorated one after another so slowly that neither I nor my relatives even noticed. I got along in school and at home fairly well because I learned, unconsciously, to *see* everything that was being said. I had to be extremely attentive, always careful to turn my head toward the speaker. I didn't realize myself how my skills improved, and how much energy that kind of constant close attention demanded. If someone spoke behind my back so that I couldn't see them, I didn't know that I was being spoken to. It was assumed that I was absent-minded.

I eventually forgot how much a human being normally can hear. Maybe my auditory nerves had never really functioned normally. It's like having sat reading without noticing that the room has grown dark little by little. Then someone enters the room, turns the light on and wonders how the other person has been able to read in such darkness.

I'm sure my family and teachers sensed something—and perhaps I sensed something myself, too. But at that time, right after the war, not much was known about disabilities, and hearing impairments were not very well understood. Disability was something to be ashamed of, something one should not have. Another issue was that my grandfather was one of the most distinguished persons in our community, a Member of Parliament and a member of the town council. As his granddaughter, I wore protective armor around me; who would dare to criticize me or examine my hearing? I got A's on exams and was always the best in my class. When someone succeeded as well as I did, she was left in peace.

When I moved from our familiar hometown to Helsinki to study, I started to realize how little I actually heard. In new situations, among new people, lipreading was impossible. When I went back home during Christmas break, my ears were humming, and I was disappointed because old familiar records didn't sound like they used to. I had to bend close to the radio to hear anything, and I could hardly talk on the telephone at all any more.

When I returned to Helsinki I went to the Student Health Center. The young doctor was stunned to find out how little I heard. He sent me to an ear specialist who told me my real situation: my auditory nerves would continue to deteriorate, and I would lose even the remaining hearing I still had.

From that visit on I started to fight for my adjustment, and that fight has not yet ended. It took nearly two years before I could admit to myself that I didn't hear. It was paralyzing when all the possibilities in life seemed to be closed. Where was a field of study where hearing was not needed? Where was the profession in which one could get by without hearing? My thoughts were in such complete chaos that I couldn't put them in order.

On the outside I still tried to pass for a hearing person. I admitted only that I "heard a bit badly," and it's not easy to get rid of that attitude. The effort to play a hearing role was tiring and used up a lot of energy that I could have used for other purposes.

Then I met Jukka. I couldn't pretend to hear very long with him. He saw the situation realistically and told me straight that my attitude was wrong. I had to live honestly as I was, and I had to fight to open up the possibilities that existed for me.

But I didn't have the strength to fight. Not for a long time.

"I can't," I said, but Jukka said, "Yes, you can." And I could. I could do a lot that I hadn't known before, and I couldn't have done it without Jukka. Little by little I started to grow out of my shell.

Gradually, after several years, I began to admit to myself that I didn't hear. Then it was time to admit it to others, and that was even more difficult. And not only did I have to admit that I heard badly, but I had to tell it exactly as it was.

How much easier it is to say "I hear badly" than "I am deaf." Often the line between these two is so vague that one can choose to take one way or the other. My choice took ten years, and it was my luck that I chose to say "I am deaf," because when I did that I found a new world.

In the deaf world, everybody speaks with hands and heart and with the whole person. When I learned to speak with my hands, I was freed from the fears that had prevented me from expressing myself. I could joke and laugh and be happy because I understood everything that was being said, and from the gestures I also learned to understand what the speaker was like. It was not until then that I realized how many different kinds of people there are in the world. How could I really have seen before, when I was painfully concentrating only on lips *sign!*

and their movements, which don't reveal anything about the speaker?

I had lived for so long with my scraps of hearing that this new world was like a wonderful liberation for me. I was accepted straightaway, immediately, among deaf people. There were many kinds of possibilities for me, possibilities that I had always longed for, but which weren't available among the hearing world. I was with people who had the same kinds of capacities that I did; they were not disabled, and I was not disabled among them.

No, Mrs. Somebody, I don't need help, thank you. I get by quite well in this new country, and after you've known me a while, you will see that for yourself.

why accepted? true fo right away? any "journey" to a new place!?

p. 12 journey metaphor not overdone, but p 14 obviously journey to acceptance of deafness)

TELEGRAMS

T he environment already looks more familiar, and I'm beginning to feel that we're not so far on the other side of the world after all, despite how we felt in the beginning. There are letters from friends, relatives, and acquaintances. They feel much closer than ever before, and even the distant ones become closer.

Besides, somewhere on this island there must be the deaf world. It must be different from the one I'm used to in my country, but still familiar to me, because sign language doesn't know boundaries even though the signs are different in each country.

"Near the department store there's a deaf man selling newspapers," Jukka tells me one day when he comes home for lunch. Besides the newspaper twice a week, Jukka is my only information source.

"How do you know, are you sure?" I ask. But at the same time I remember the man who sits behind cardboard containers outside the Minvielle & Chastanet department store, known as the M.K.C., on Bridge Street. On top of the containers there is a pile of newspapers. The man always wears a woolen cap in spite of the summer heat, as do many other youngsters on the island.

I remember the coin incident. Last time I bought the island newspaper from the man, I also wanted to buy the Barbados paper. I looked up the prices for the papers and dug out the needed coins. But no, it was not enough. I had forgotten that they have a different currency on Barbados. The salesman took coins from his pocket, gestured, and showed how many and what kinds of coins I still had to give him. I imagined that he showed things visually this way for me because he noticed that I didn't hear. But it was because he was deaf himself!

At the end of November I saw in *The Voice of St. Lucia* paper the headline

"Sign Language." It left me shaken, as any familiar name or topic in the newspaper always does.

"The teacher of the deaf, Clyde Vincent, is starting sign language lessons. The lessons will be held Monday evenings at the school for the deaf in the St. John's Ambulance Building. Sign language is a unique language, comprised of movements of hands and fingers and facial expressions, which is used when communicating with a deaf person. Mr. Vincent tells us that everybody is welcome to his lessons, especially parents of deaf children."

That was a way for me to get into the deaf world in St. Lucia! Socializing doesn't happen instantly, I know that; but one has to start somewhere.

On Monday evening we drive to the school for the deaf. Jukka comes along because I need him, Keke, or Joppe once in a while to interpret for me. The situation is new, I don't know enough English yet, and I can't read it from the lips. When Jukka is speaking English, I understand almost everything because I'm so used to his lip movements. Besides, Jukka takes care that he's speaking toward me, even when he's talking to somebody else.

We wait in the school yard because we're not yet used to the island time. We go to parties at the time printed on the invitation, only to find out that the hosts are not yet prepared to receive us. The other guests start arriving after an hour or so.

The palms on the mountain slopes are dimly turquoise. It is five-thirty and the sun is setting. The warm afternoon changes all of a sudden into a cooler darkness. But just before the sun finally sets behind the mountains, a man with a beard drives his motor bike into the yard. He has a rucksack; he wears a checked shirt and corduroy jeans. Is he the American teacher for the deaf?

We go in, and Jukka asks, "Are you Clyde Vincent?"

Jukka repeats his question, and the man nods. He walks rapidly into the office behind the classroom, takes a pen and paper from his drawer, turns the fan on, opens the shades, and starts writing very fast. Then Jukka writes, Clyde writes, Jukka writes, and I start to understand what is meant by "writing with your pen on fire." Many pieces of paper get filled up, and finally I realize that this bearded teacher is deaf. Jukka must have seen it already at the door, because his mouth movements were especially clear when he repeatedly asked the man's name.

I have a lot to learn from Clyde. How easily he took up his pen and paper. In the way he started his writing there was power, which at once forced the other person to reply by writing.

Other people are arriving. The teacher takes up a primitive blackboard, folding chairs are brought from somewhere, and the lesson starts. The fan is buzzing on the ceiling. I am suffering from the draft even though it's warm, because I am not yet used to the fact that over here all possible windows are always open.

The shelf next to the roughly made blackboard keeps falling down and spilling the sponge and crayons on the floor. Clyde writes on the board, signs, gives written pieces of paper to the hearing people in the class. We could just as well be attending a sign language course in Finland. We learn what sign language is, what different kinds there are, how to communicate with a deaf person. Everything is familiar to me except that the signs in this American Sign Language are very different from Finnish signs.

"Book," "rain," and "to see," for example, are completely similar: they describe clearly opening the book, the falling of raindrops, and looking. But if I use the Finnish sign "to remember," it means "dumb" in this language, and "sister" means "friend."

The teacher shows visually what the universal language of deaf people is like: facial expressions, gestures, and hand movements that can't be exactly translated into spoken language. They are simply sign language. Very often one sign equals a whole spoken sentence. Many expressions are so funny and so strikingly to the point that we laugh aloud. We laugh even more when one person tries to fingerspell and form signs with hands that don't want to bend into the required positions.

All of a sudden I get the same pleasure and sense of enjoyment that I always get among deaf people. I look at Jukka, who sits in the back and tries to sign. He is no beginner. He's very proud because he signs to me at home every morning "half a cup of coffee" because, half asleep, I just can't follow the small movements of the lips. Jukka doesn't hide his light under a bushel; at parties he tells everybody the story of his "half a cup." This way he has spread information about sign language to people who otherwise never would have learned about the deaf and their language. Many people have difficulty even imaging a person with

[handwritten margin note: most of us will be disabled by the time we die]

[handwritten margin note: could be anyone]

a disability—although any of these flawless ones could just as well lose their hearing and experience the same difficulties I'm going through now.

Clyde looks at me as if at a hearing person. After the lesson I go to him and speak with my hands: "I deaf same you."

These signs I know, and I don't need to prattle long. It's like sending a telegram.

Clyde looks surprised. All of a sudden I feel I have stepped over an unseen line into his world, and he has accepted me. But I'm still a stranger, because Clyde picks up his pen and paper again. He realizes that we don't have the same sign language.

I show Clyde the Finnish Sign Language dictionary that I've brought along. He looks at the pictures and the Finnish words below them and then writes, "I'd like to learn your sign language. Can you translate twenty pages for me for next Monday, and then the next twenty pages for the following Monday?"

I try to write my answer: there are about four thousand signs in the book, and I don't know more than about two thousand of them myself—the ones I had to study to get my sign language instructor's certificate.

But Clyde writes determinedly, "I know American Sign Language so well that it's easy for me to acquire a new sign language."

Okay. We shall see which one of us will learn the other one's sign language faster. I laugh as I write this. I challenge him to a contest, although I know already that I will lose. I've learned sign language as an adult, haven't I, but for Clyde it is his first language, his mother tongue in which he can express himself completely. Also, there are so many common elements in different sign languages that one who knows sign language well is able to change it so that any foreign deaf person can understand it.

"My parents are deaf. There are five of us children, all of us deaf."

I see! Clyde grew up with sign language as his first language. In addition, he writes good English. The community must have been horrified at the deaf family without realizing that they were a normal family. Only their language was different from that of the neighbors. *[handwritten margin note: probably true]*

Now that I have my contact with the deaf, I feel that my life on the island has some significance to it. It's now that I can completely settle down.

"What did you tell Clyde about me?" I ask Jukka on our way home.

"I told him that you have a degree in education and that you have a certificate in sign language instruction. Clyde said that you're welcome to teach at his school. Help is needed there."

"Oh heavens. I don't have any experience in teaching deaf children, only theoretical information."

"You have more knowledge about the deaf and their problems than many other people over here. You have worked at the Deaf Association and created courses for deaf adults."

"Yes, but . . ."

Once again Jukka has more trust in my abilities than I do myself. Maybe he's right, as he's always been before. But first I have to learn American Sign Language. We'll see after that . . .

what do you think of her family?

because of this, still be "thrust" into the culture

DEAF SCHOOL

The following week Clyde invites me to Open Door Day at the school for the deaf. I arrive early so that I have time to meet Clyde and his students before the other guests arrive. Four pupils have come to school for the model lesson. One of the boys is about a head taller than the others. The only girl in the group has on a nice blue and white dress and a mysterious Mona Lisa smile. The pupils are about 12 or 13 years old. Clyde calls them "my children," and they do look like children still.

"This is Kenneth." Clyde makes the introduction, his right hand forming the letter K on the forehead. Victor: the forefinger and middle finger in V-position on the forehead. Joseph, the tall boy: the little finger draws a letter J on the forehead. Theresa: a letter T on the cheek near the chin.

"Is your name Ruth?" Clyde asks.

"No, *R-a-i-j-a.*" I spell my name with the hand alphabet; *i-j* is difficult, it often becomes a *y.* Even more difficult is our last name, Nieminen. It has *i, e, m* and *n* in a strange combination that is difficult for an English speaker.

Clyde puts his hand in R-position on the left side of his chest. Maybe it's just a randomly chosen place, but Clyde has created my name sign!

People begin arriving at the school: sisters from the Catholic St. Joseph School, teachers and students from the Anglican school next door, students from the Morne Teacher Training College, parents and relatives of the deaf pupils.

In the dim hallway the ladies from the Society for the Deaf are selling guava jam, Christmas cards, and crocheted tablecloths. The society is not "of the deaf" but "for the deaf," a benevolent organization. The parents of the children in the school are members of the society—they are the most educated and active among the parents of deaf children.

Two American teachers started the school two years ago with help from the Society for the Deaf. I don't know who took the initiative. Now Clyde teaches small children under ten years of age in the mornings and older children in the afternoons. Clyde is a member of the U.S. Peace Corps; he gets room and board, but no salary.

In the mornings there's also an audiologist working at the school whom the government pays half a day's salary. Otherwise the government gives very little support to the school. St. Lucia has been an independent member country in the British Commonwealth for only eight years. There are so many things that the small republic has to accomplish that deaf education is not yet on the list of priorities.

"We need children, teachers, teaching materials," one paper on the school wall says. There are 110,000 inhabitants on St. Lucia. The society knows of sixty school-age deaf children. There are twenty-three children in the school now.

I feel as though I'm in my element when I'm in this school. This is my world. The deaf pupils show me their notebooks and handiwork. Clyde gives a model lesson with his pupils.

"Victor, get a book," Clyde signs.

Victor gets the book, and the spectators stare in wonder. "Look now," Clyde wants to say, "these children can be talked to, they understand what I say with my hands even though they don't hear speech. They can be taught!"

surprise at what deaf people can do - shows their ignorance

deaf school feels more like home - what small groups? would make Mor feel this way

OBLIGATIONS IN SOCIAL CIRCLES

[handwritten notes: frustration of understood / lack of understood / + unfamiliar environment ✱ party bad experience — what should we do to include people more?]

Mrs. X has called and asked, "Can your wife come to my cocktail party even though she doesn't hear?" Jukka tells me one day.

This is one more frustrating moment when I remember that the hearing impairment exists and that people don't understand it at all.

On the other hand, however, maybe Mrs. X only wanted to save me from a depressing experience.

I stand with a glass in my hand. I am annoyed and grow angrier every moment. I should smile politely, but my smile is already anything but natural.

Mouths keep moving; everybody laughs. I don't know any more frustrating situation than that people are laughing, and I don't know why. It seems odd if I am serious alone, but what could I laugh about?

I can laugh, too, and joke, talk, and discuss, if only they knew. I am just like any other person. I remember the evening before I left for the island, after the committee meeting of the Deaf Magazine in the Red Hat restaurant with Runo, Aura, Rea, and Jarmo. Red farewell carnations were glowing on the table in warm candlelight, and there was still enough light for us to talk. But now, the ice cubes in the glass feel cold in my fingers. Coldness spreads and makes me numb. I'd like to throw the glass to the floor and run away, but at the same time I would run away from Jukka. Once in a while I must have the strength to be with him on these occasions—luckily not too often.

Jukka helps whenever he gets a chance, but he can't fill every moment. He tells me what they laughed about, I also try to laugh, but all the others have already laughed and are looking at me—I mustn't roar with laughter alone.

[handwritten notes: your reac to this? (same hearing couples) partners support one another]

But sometimes it can happen like this: I notice that there's an exotic-looking woman standing in front of me; maybe she is Japanese.

"Mmmmmmmm," she says.

"I'm sorry, but I cannot hear what you say. I cannot read English from the lips," I say tiredly, and wait for the woman to go away. Most people do, because they are afraid of communication problems. But this woman won't give up.

"Mmmmm live mmm?" A wave of her hand that I automatically understand to mean "here." Her facial expression tells me that she is asking something.

"Yes, we do live here; we're staying two years." I'm spirited already.

"Where are you from?" I ask in my turn.

"C . . N . . . D?" I have to make several guesses before I interpret the sounds that I can't read. Grenada? Greenland? Canada?

Canada is the right answer. The woman is shivering, and I understand that she wants to show me that it's cold in Canada.

"I'm from Finland, and it's cold there, too." It's almost as if I had met a countryman. In the end, how little is needed. But people don't understand even that little, and they don't offer it. They don't want to bother with it.

a little effort is all that's needed

do you make it here?

do your Int. students

ENCOUNTER ON THE SQUARE

It's always summer here, and I don't notice that Christmas is getting close. In the stores, black hams are hanging in the heat of the sun—they might be covered with pitch. In the window of the M.K.C. department store a snowman is staring with black eyes. It seems odd to see it under the tropical sun. One might be afraid it would melt . . . but of course it's made of cotton. Children crowd around the toy windows, just as in any other town before Christmas.

We read in the paper that stores are open in the evenings because of Christmas. We drive into town one evening, but it's raining, and the streets are empty, and the doors of the stores are shut tight. There are mail sacks in front of the post office—no, they're dogs; sleeping on the sidewalk like chilled bundles.

The following evening the shops are open, but all of a sudden the electricity goes off. The doors quickly close, and people wander confused in the dark streets.

But before Christmas there will be an evening when it's not raining and the lights stay on, and that's when there's a lively bustle in the streets and stores. Little boys are winding in and out of the streets, throwing firecrackers in the middle of the crowd and causing a startled uproar of smoke and hissing. In front of the Bata shoe store a man with a scarf on his head sits on the pavement rhythmically beating a tin can. Somebody is moving to the rhythm. Stores, streets, and cinemas are flooded with people moving about.

We buy Keke a chess game and Joppe a small Japanese radio. Very little merchandise is available, but it's relaxing to shop when the head isn't spinning around because of too many things. Even plastic bags are just now finding their way onto the island.

A few days before Christmas the Port Office holds its Christmas party. The Ministry of Communication, Works, and Labor and the Port Authority are situated in an old English military barracks with walls half a meter thick. The building was supposed to be torn down and a new concrete office building constructed, but Jukka arrived just in time to save the beautiful, historic building. Its thick walls make it ideal for this climate.

We climb up steep wooden stairs to the second floor. At the door we meet a polite gentleman in a white uniform. He is Sir Charles Bousquet, the chief pilot of the port, who recently was knighted by the British queen. Port Director Monplaisir, bookkeeper Daniel, the operations manager Peter Paul . . . I'll surely get to know all these people better later on.

Jukka's secretary Maureen Moffat brings plates of food for us. The women in the office have prepared the food at home, and according to St. Lucia custom, food is ladled straight onto the plates. Maureen is an Englishwoman who has married a man from St. Lucia and lives on the island now. Mr. Moffat is a reporter for the St. Lucia radio station.

I don't have time to get tired or frustrated, because after we eat, we must dance, according to the local custom. Here one enters into the spirit of dance completely; talking to your dancing partner is not appropriate. It's easy to dance with the St. Lucia people: I look at my partner, and move as he does, and the rhythm draws us into the dance.

Doubtful Christmas greetings are arriving from our home country. "We have snow and cold here; you are there in the warmth. I wonder if you have Christmas over there at all . . ."

Of course we have Christmas. Jukka has bought a Christmas tree, a sweet-smelling tamarack. When the tree is brought in in the morning, we can smell the fine aromas of brush and incense. The tree is so beautiful that we hardly dare hang any trinkets on it. Everywhere outside, the man-size poinsettias are in bloom—the same as we get at home in small flowerpots labeled "Christmas Star."

Zenia presents her packages shyly, and we find two souvenirs. They get a special place on a shelf. Zenia receives food from us for Christmas, and a colorful towel that Keke and Joppe found for her.

By midday Zenia has left, the Christmas tree is in its place, mutton steak is baking in the oven, and Keke is frying special spiced chicken. We phone our family at home. In Finland they are farther ahead in their Christmas celebrations; they have already had their Christmas dinner and are waiting for Santa Claus to arrive. Our telephone call comes as a surprise to Jukka's sister Leena and her family, because everyone thought we had moved to some unknown faraway place and would never be heard from again.

We celebrate as Finnish a Christmas Eve as possible. We eat in the kitchen by candlelight, but first Keke reads the Christmas Gospel from his English Bible. I can see he reads it beautifully; we all have a nice peaceful feeling.

"Glory to God in the highest, and on earth peace, good will toward men . . ."

After that Eve, Christmas peace is all gone. We meet local people and visitors who have arrived on the island from different parts of the world. Back home in Finland, a foreigner was a rare thing; here we meet people from the north, south, east, and west every day. I try to get acquainted with these people by looking closely at their way of speaking, their behavior, and their expressions, but how interesting it would be to hear what they say!

As the New Year gets close I am worn out from the stifling heat, the bustle, and the intense concentration. I remember what our friend Lasse Terho, who had worked in tropical countries, told us before we left: "Your time on the island will be tiring for you, Raija. Do remember that!"

He was right. I told Jukka, "Let's not go anywhere for a couple of weeks. I don't understand why I'm so tired. I don't have as much energy here as I do in Finland."

"The same goes for me," Jukka says. "It's this language. Sometimes I feel my brains are bursting with all the new words. Each evening I'm completely exhausted from speaking English all day long."

And for two weeks Jukka refuses all invitations so that I have time to pull myself together and gather energy to be polite, to appear interested, even though I don't have the faintest idea what people are talking about. I have just strength enough to concentrate on following the lip movements; I try to participate somehow.

But first the New Year! On New Year's Eve when it's getting close to midnight, the inhabitants dress in their best. White dress collars, hats, shirts, and gloves gleam in the dim, wet streets as people walk to the Catholic church for midnight mass, their black books under their arms, or to services at the Baptist or Adventist churches. The Catholic cathedral on the square is full of people. Up on the altar, thin candles are flickering; in front of the Virgin Mary there are dozens of them. The priest in his white chasuble is so far away that I can't even see his lips, but the atmosphere breathes out into the street through the open doors. We are standing on the street, but I am overwhelmed by the warm, dusky atmosphere of the cathedral.

Not until the mass is over at two o'clock in the morning do people start celebrating the changing of the year. We drive up the mountain to the big house of our Indian friend. There are a lot of people holding glasses in their hands or dancing, but the lighting is so dim that the only thing I can sense is the smell of the antimosquito smoke and the cool, wet wind that blows through the house.

On New Year's Day Columbus Square has changed into a busy marketplace, with boards and corrugated-metal market stands crammed in next to each other on all sides of the square. For four days and four nights people crowd the alleyways in the midst of the smells of coconut oil, coal-pot smoke, and fried fish balls. In the stalls, chicken legs and flying fish, rolled in flour, are fried in pots over hot coals. Ice cream machines hum continuously.

We move with the tightly packed human mass. The hem of my long skirt drags in the mud, and I hang onto Jukka's arm so I won't lose him. The ancient samantrees on the square form a cover through which the air can hardly move. Keke and Joppe have gone their own ways. They stay near us less and less; they're starting to lead their own lives. It occurs to me that in a few months Keke will go back to Finland to go to school, but I push the thought quickly to the back of my mind.

"Hello!" somebody shouts from a stall.

"That's Abraham Biscombe over there," says Jukka. "He works at the Ministry of Communication, Works, and Labor. Every time I pass his room at the Port Office he greets me."

"What do you want to have ? It's my treat," Abraham says.

I tell him I want coffee, because the night is wet and cool with rain. Everyone is surprised—nobody drinks coffee at Columbus Square on New Year's.

After that we stop frequently, and I'm surprised how many people Jukka already knows over here: port workers, truck drivers and their bosses, ministry workers, and other government workers.

We're treated to beer and ice cream, but just as often, Jukka digs out his wallet and pays.

"How many children do you have?" is the first thing we ask families that we meet.

"Well, with this wife one and five with other women . . ."

Although they speak with pride, we stop asking about children.

The atmosphere on the Square is cheerful, and above all there's the constant, endless, rhythmic music that thumps to the very marrow of my bones and makes my body sway while my knees keep time—like all the other people on the Square.

All of a sudden I feel that someone is touching me. A boy is standing in front of me—asking for a coin?

But the boy is only staring at me; he has an open look and a slightly timid smile; his blue-gray shirt is clean and ironed. When I still don't show any sign of recognition, the boy puts his right hand shyly on his left collarbone in the R-position.

My name sign! It's the name Clyde gave me at school during Open Door Day. This boy is one of Clyde's students, then, isn't he? Maybe Kenneth? He must be Kenneth. I try out the letter K on my forehead. The boy nods and smiles happily.

How in the world did the boy know me in the crowded Square and even remember my name?

I get stage fright. What will I sign to him? I don't yet know the sign language these children use. I feel as if I were a beginner who thinks that you have to know exactly the correct signs to be able to talk with a deaf person.

Jukka gives the boy a dollar bill from his wallet, but I can't give him anything, although he's looking at me as if I'm a friend he's happy to have found.

In the car on the way home I feel that this encounter in the Square has wiped away all the other experiences during the Christmas season. All I can see is the little boy in front of me making my name sign. It was like the emblem of a secret brotherhood in the crowded Square.

I have to do something on my own for these children. Kenneth and the other children don't need my pity any more than I need pity from other people, but I can try to give them something from myself and at the same time find a new meaning for my stay here. Maybe everything I've experienced so far, all the depressing and frustrating experiences but also the inspiring and encouraging ones, have been necessary so that, in my turn, I can help others. But I also understand that one person alone can't accomplish very much, no matter how hard she tries. Everybody can do only her own share, whether the result turns out to be small or a bit bigger, beautiful or entirely invisible.

SMALL VISITORS

We have to move out of Vigie because the Rogerses are coming to the island and want to use their cottage. We move in early January on a glowing sunny day. Near the new house the blue sea and a golden-yellow beach can be seen behind the palms and the red bougainvilleas.

The rainy season is over, and the sky is cloudless almost all day; in the afternoons, rain clouds move down from the mountains. They bring enough showers for Nature to stay green.

Our home is in the Sunny Acres area, along the Cap Estate road leading to the north end of the island. Our landlord, Victor Archer, is a retired teacher from the West Indies University. He lives with his wife a little way up the slope.

Regular pest extermination has not been done in this house as it was in our Vigie house, so now I have to handle the hardships and difficulties of the tropics that I prepared for so well when I left Finland!

Along the walls and floors of the house, rows of small ants run fast. They climb up my feet, and in an instant they've attacked the sugar and cookies on the table. In the mornings the kitchen floor is full of sawdust, and on the third morning I realize that there are mice living in the cupboards. New spiderwebs appear each day on the ceiling, in corners, and on lamps. Green lizards swarm on the railing of the balcony and the iron bars of the windows. Millipedes wind along the bedroom floor. One evening there's a huge slug lying on the bathroom shelf on top of the toothpaste—it's at least fifteen centimeters long and two wide!

Sometimes I take a spray bottle and start spraying into the midst of the ant army, but somehow I can't continue because they're so touchingly diligent and energetic. They drag along huge brown creatures with long antennae—cockroaches! Even dead these are dreadful. I almost shriek when a five-centimeter-long cockroach wheels along the floor or wall straight toward me. I pick up my shoe and end its run.

I feel sorry for ants and lizards, but I have to get an exterminator, who comes with a mask covering his head, to spray poison all through the house. I have to empty the cupboards again—and I just got them arranged. The next day it's quiet. There are dead cockroaches on the floor that have crept from their hiding places during the night. No ants are in sight, and there's no sawdust on the kitchen floor. After a few days, the lizards come back, after two months the cockroaches return, but right behind them comes the masked man with his poison spray.

Poisonous snakes live on the tops of the mountains, and there are big poisonous spiders living on the island, but they are quite rare. I notice that I am too well prepared. The expensive disinfectants, poisons, and medicines grow moldy in their plastic boxes in the cupboards. When I get the flu for the first time, Dr. King takes a glance at my medicines and says that he'll prescribe something more potent for me.

We now have a big garden, and we lure Anderson here from Vigie to look after it. He brings his all-purpose tool: a huge, fierce-looking jungle knife. With that he gets everything done in the garden: cutting the grass, cutting branches, turning the soil. With that same knife he can also split coconuts, slice meat, and clean fish.

There are coconut trees, banana trees, papaya trees, okra bushes, and a Royal Poinciana (also called a flamboyant tree) growing in the garden. The garden is constantly changing. Anderson plants hibiscus bushes and brings some packets of seeds: lettuce, radish, cucumber. He asks me what is written on each packet, and after that he throws the seeds into the soil. He also plants tomatoes, which I water in the evening at sunset. It's a nice job because I don't want to work in the garden in the heat of the afternoon. Anderson does that, with sweat dripping down his shiny face.

Anderson nails sticks to the pole on the balcony and forces the Virginia creeper to grow along them, so that it will give us shade against the severest heat. Before long the garden produces pumpkins and yellow-green tomatoes, which we wrap in paper and put on the shelf of the vegetable closet next to the papayas ripening in paper bags. Outside, fruit would ripen too fast, become soft and collapse in our hands.

"When do you think you will marry Zenia?" Jukka asks Anderson.

"I don't quite know, sir. If I marry Zenia, I have to look after her four children."

Four children! No wonder Zenia is often so tired in the afternoons that she rests her head on the table.

One morning Zenia stands at the door looking shy and points to her stomach. "Baby."

I don't know what to say. One more child can't lower Zenia's standard of living any further, and this society appreciates a woman who has many children. So that's why Zenia is happy and proud. She doesn't know anything about newspaper articles saying that too many children are born on the island. Over half of the inhabitants are now children. Educational and employment problems therefore are great.

"Have you seen the doctor yet?"

"I am only in the fifth month," Zenia says happily.

The boys go to school. Castries Comprehensive Secondary School has been recommended to us. It was built with help from the Canadians and has Canadian teachers. The headmaster is local and doesn't like to take white students— they'll only bring trouble . . . Jukka assures him that the boys will surely behave well, and so the headmaster agrees to take them.

The first days in school are a trial for the boys. There are less than ten white students in the school; they are in the minority and can feel it in many ways. Joppe, especially, has difficulties. He knows very little English, and he wants to succeed in everything. The boys don't even have school uniforms.

Well, that's easy to take care of. We go to town to the J.Q. Charles store and buy black pants, black shoes, and white jacket-like shirts for the boys.

Fortunately the school is very close by, so the boys don't need to walk a long way in the afternoon in the burning sun. Jukka buys a Mirror sailboat for the boys to cheer them up, and we start visiting the Reduit Beach Yacht Club on weekends.

One day when I come home from town I see four dark boys sitting on the living room couch. On the table are glasses of juice with lots of ice, and the red light on the record player is glowing. I feel a vibration that almost splits my head open. Whenever I move, four pairs of eyes follow me closely, critically.

A wrinkled piece of paper on the table explains everything: "I intend to visit your home this afternoon. I want to meet your mother."

Of course I'm flattered that the reason for this visit is me.

In the living room, I talk to Keke, watching closely what he says; in my turn I answer him. When the visitors are gone, Keke brings the glasses to the kitchen.

"The boys said that you do so hear!" he explains, looking amused.

"Yes, I do hear well with my eyes."

I feel good. Keke has told his mates about my hearing impairment, relevantly and without shame.

From that day on, one of the boys, John Eugene, comes over every day and watches me and Jukka closely. John Eugene is curious; he wants to find out about the white mother and father and about the white family. But after a while he stops staring. We are no longer his white schoolmate's white family, but simply his schoolmate's family.

The town streets become familiar to me, and I begin to feel at home here. But the taxi drivers wave, wanting to give me a ride; little boys put out their hands to beg for money, or an old wrinkled woman, almost blind, repeats in front of me "Penny, penny."

I want to say, "I'm one of you, I live here. I'm not an American tourist whose money you ask for so eagerly."

Sometimes in the evening I cover my fair hair with a scarf, take a paper bag in my hand and walk along the dark streets to the bakery. I work myself up to my turn at the counter and make sure that I get fifteen fresh, crisp, ten-cent breads. Nobody is looking at me; for a moment I'm one of them.

The sun shines hot, toasting our faces and limbs almost as dark as those of the islanders.

Music and rhythm fill us because they're part of life here. Our muscles relax, we move and dance like our friends. Rhythms roll inside me, under my chestbone and through all my bones as if they're being pounded by the powerful beat.

When Abraham and his wife Monica come to visit, we sit quietly at first. I

— 34 —

offer drinks and salted peanuts. Jukka puts a calypso record on. I look at Abraham's dark body, swaying before me. In a moment the rhythm overtakes me and I move as if I am his mirror image. There's no more black or white, only four happy people in the swing of a dance. If it could always be like this, we all could live in one world—there would be no black or white, there would be no deaf or hearing. We all would hold the keys to the one world we all would inhabit.

In the evenings we walk along Jeremie Street and enjoy its busy life. I think of the tourists who come here and see only swimming pools, the sun, and the water. In their eagerness to soak up the sun, they forget they're wearing beach clothes when they walk along the main street and shop at supermarkets. They don't understand that they offend local custom by dressing that way.

Jeremie Street starts at the marketplace. Along it are small shops and bars that have received "a licence to sell intoxicating drinks," as it says on the sign above the broad doorway. The shop where I buy my rice is open even in the evenings. The woman weighs rice and flour from dawn until dusk and eats her meals sitting behind the counter. There are bags full of flour and brown sugar and boxes of dried cod. On the shelf are milk powder, soap, matches, and canned meat.

At the marketplace, the mango seller sits under the clock. His fruit is partly in the basket, partly on the muddy street. It almost always rains enough for the streets and the marketplace to be muddy. After a hot day the coconut shells and the remains of the fruit stink in the mud.

Far away are the cities bathed in neon lights. On Jeremie Street, in the evenings, you see people only as vague figures in the dark or in the dim light that shines from the doors of shops and saloons. The rental housing into which people have moved from the countryside lines the street. I'm sure there are a lot of sounds in the street; I can guess from the busy bustle.

Men sit in the small square under the flamboyant trees. I wonder if they're the same men at night as during the day. Some of them play dominoes or checkers. All day and all night the street sellers sit in their places with their trays of fruit and candy. Someone has brought out a table and is selling fried chicken legs and small cakes to passersby. Yellow corncobs fry over the coal pots.

Hands are raised to greet us. Jukka is called "the chief."

"I like you because you have such a calm face." A man walks beside Jukka and talks. These people talk with their hands, so I don't get as bored looking at them as I would if I had to concentrate on their lips.

Jukka treats everybody in a straightforward way, but these people are themselves straightforward and say what they think. Someone grabs Jukka's hand.

"I like that you walk here along our street. What can I treat you to?"

We go inside through the hanging plastic strips into the violet light of the saloon. We sit beside the bar counter under the fan and drink cold beer. It makes me sweat. Jukka's shirt gleams white against his suntanned skin.

A man in a cap approaches us carrying a bag. He shakes our hands. I tug at Jukka's sleeve.

"Who is he, what is he saying?"

"He just wanted to say hello to us."

Jukka has to tell everybody where we're from: a small, poor country far away to the north. People don't know anything about Finland except that they don't have anything against our country and that it must be cold because it's located so far to the north. They ask how we like their island, and they're satisfied when we tell them that we're happy here. Everybody wants us to enjoy ourselves.

I guess that's why we sometimes find a bag of juicy seedless grapefruit, wrinkled lemons, or earthy forked yams outside our door in the mornings. Sometimes someone brings a heavy, red-eye perch, green oranges or honey, or fragrant-smelling roots for our linen closet. Or Anderson stands behind the door and hands me a bag full of sweet peppers, lettuce, or flying fish that he has cleaned and marinated.

Keke and Joppe munch fruit, and their cheeks get rounder. They can eat nearly twenty bananas and five grapefruit in one day!

If we need something special or if something in the house needs repair work, we get help from the port. Simon Bartholomew, the chief of the repair shop, comes with his helpers and their tools. They fix what's broken in a wink and then have coffee on the balcony. Peter Paul, the inspector for cargo-handling, knows what goods and services are available and where to get them. Little by little, Peter Paul becomes very important to us. At the port he is Jukka's right hand. Maureen Moffat is the only secretary who can keep up with Jukka.

She also takes care of my telephone needs, phoning for a doctor's appointment and so on because I can't use the phone. Life starts to settle down into a comfortable rut.

we need to get comfortable before taking new risks? deaf school involvement will come soon

BY THE SHORE
OF THE
SAPPHIRE SEA

Mango trees are starting to bloom. Their sweet smell is everywhere. I fear that Keke will become sick because he is so allergic to pollen. The mango blooms can't be seen, they only smell, but soon there's another tree in bloom that makes the whole scene look like an apple orchard. It's called the apple-bloom cassia. On the shore in the midst of the coconut palms, the apple-bloom tree's pink flowers shine against the blue sky. How beautiful the tropical winter is!

The sun sets in the evening to the left of the lighthouse. The palm fronds reflect against the bright red sky, darker and darker until only black fanlike silhouettes can be seen against the glow of color. The night-blue starts to grow darker on the skyline, and more and more stars begin to shine. Just before sunset the lizards run around the balcony rail, and the air is full of zigzagging bats. The light from the lighthouse cuts through the night sky all the more brightly, gleaming on the shiny palm leaves. The wonderful performance of the sunset takes about an hour. After the dark, starry night, the morning is glowing and fresh.

I sit on the balcony and write to Aino Viitala back home: "I'm sure you'd love to be here on a day like this. The sky is blue, palms are swaying, it's warm, but a fresh wind is blowing."

Aino is a farmer's wife on a big northern farm and is active in cultural activities at the Deaf Association. How she would love all this beauty.

Just after I mail my letter, I get a letter from my friend Kaisu Korhonen. "Aino fell ill in the late fall. She was sometimes in the hospital, and sometimes at home. Because she was always so interested in different countries, I sent her a part of your letter to me in which you told about the life on the island. She was very interested and filled with wonder.

"Alas, she would have been very interested in your new letter, too, about all this color and warmth, in the midst of this death-silent Finnish nature of ours which always makes us so reserved. Night frost can appear even in the middle of the bright summer, and what gets frostbitten does not get renewed.

"Aino is dead."

Aino is dead. No, it can't be true, I don't want it to be true. I cry and cry, over everything—that I have only a few good friends and I have now lost one, a fine and wonderful person whom I couldn't even visit during her last days. At this moment I feel achingly how far away from home we really are.

Through my tears I see the palms, the sea, and the white clouds in the sky, and I remember the verses from Kaisu's letter:

> White sails of clouds
> By the shore of the sapphire sea,
> In the swing of the ebb and tide
> The heart has its sweet bed.

LEARN THE LESSON

On this island I finally have to learn my lesson, and in the end it happens in a very simple way.

When I go to the supermarket a kilometer away, I walk. When I go shopping in town, I use the buses traveling between the Gros Islet fishing village and the town. But almost always before the bus comes or before I have had time to walk even a hundred meters, a car stops, and the driver offers me a ride. People have to travel long distances out here to go to work or to school. The general custom is for drivers to offer a ride whenever they can. Even Jukka, when he drives to work in the morning, carries a full load of students in their pretty school uniforms: blue, green, red, and purple skirts, dark slacks, white, blue, or yellow blouses—every school has its own colors. The girls wear their hair in small pigtails with big colorful bows. They have bright golden earrings in their ears.

Soon the drivers don't stop to offer a ride, but just point forward with a questioning look. Then I have to nod quickly. The car stops about twenty meters away. I run, shout "Hello," and push myself into an empty seat. At that point it's a good idea to say, "Sorry, I'm deaf. I can't hear what you say!" before anyone has time to ask me anything.

Some people don't say anything after that, but press their lips tightly together so they won't speak by accident. But most people won't give up.

I know what I will probably be asked. "Are you German?"

"No, I'm not German. I'm from Finland. My husband works here as General Manager for the Port Authority. We intend to stay here two years."

Sometimes when I don't feel like taking the initiative, I don't give the necessary information, but everything is usually revealed very quickly.

"Mmmmmmm?"

much can be predicted

"???"

"You do not speak English?"

I almost always can grasp the world "English" and the rest I can guess.

"Yes, I do speak English, but I am deaf. I have to read from the lips what I am being told, and that is difficult here, because English is not my mother tongue."

"Oh, I see."

Sometimes the person digs a piece of paper from the glove compartment and a pen from his pocket and tries to write while driving. After these kinds of rides I feel lighthearted.

Sometimes, when I'm in a really brave mood, I even take the initiative myself.

"How long have you been here on the island?" Or if the driver is local, I might discuss the weather. That's something to talk about at length, because the weather on the island is always abnormal. It either rains more than it has in years, or it's exceptionally cool or hot.

But although I could learn my lesson by heart, it wouldn't be enough, because too many hearing people still believe that deafness prevents me from living and working. Some matters I can change myself, but there are a lot of things that even Jukka can't do anything about. *disappointments ignorance*

We once fought really hard and lost—I didn't get a job that was suited to my education. There was somebody else who either had more work experience, although I had the higher degree, or the higher degree carried more weight—if the other person had it, not me. In the end I realized that there are always ways to make the other applicant—the one who hears well—seem better qualified for the job.

Fortunately, Jukka has furnished work for my mind and a use for the knowledge I have gathered. I've proofread his memos and helped him make speeches and write newspaper articles. I've tried to be the wife every career-minded husband needs to back him up and help him get ahead.

In the deaf world I've been able to use my knowledge and skills at full force. At the Deaf Association they needed resources badly, and as soon as I was introduced, I got lots of tasks to do. It felt wonderful. No, I didn't read piles of books,

people always realize they're deaf this?

— 41 —

write surveys, and sit many hours every week in buses on my way to exams and lectures in vain.

I met Jukka at the Student Union dances during my very first year of university. Jukka was almost through with his studies at the Commercial College and was leaving to go to sea. That's why we got engaged after dating for only two months. I did have my doubts, though. I had just seen the ear specialist and was collapsing from the news that I would eventually lose my hearing completely. It seemed impossible to think of getting married when the future was so threatening. But in Jukka's opinion, a hearing impairment was only one part of an entirety. Many other things mean much more than that.

Jukka went to sea, and I continued sorting out my crisis without his support. I wandered along the hallways from one class to another; I tried to be like all the other students. I studied German and Swedish. I kept carrying my red binder with the dividers labeled with titles like *Behaghel* and *Grammatik* and *Vogelweide*. I buttoned my cardigan in the back according to the latest fashion like all the other casual-looking women students. I sat in the smoked-filled cafe, drinking my coffee.

What nonsense the whole thing was—to sit in the classroom without hearing anything, without knowing what was going on. I had chosen the wrong subjects. I had a head for languages, but languages demand good hearing. All the other students were madly taking notes; how on earth could they make any sense of the teacher's mumbling? In big rooms the voice of the lecturer didn't even reach my ears, never mind that I wouldn't have heard the words anyway.

I borrowed notes from my friend Pirjo Vesanen, who attended the same lectures I did. Pirjo was my best support in those days. I went on with my studies because I didn't know what else to do.

The university information office seemed like a symbol of all my insecurity. It was the only place where I could even try to ask for answers to my problems—answers that I didn't get—because the office workers didn't move their lips at all.

I managed some exams, but not enough. I knew what people in my hometown would think: "She used to do well in school, but now she doesn't seem to get anywhere at all. I guess she'll just remain a high school graduate, no more." I had heard these same phrases whispered about other students.

fear of ~ not what
telling ~ understand
understand happen

To be able to pass the German course, cum laude, with honors, I had to get to the proseminar. To make it that far, a student had to pass two exams: translation and *Nacherzahlung*. This meant that the teacher read aloud a German story and you had to write it down in your own words afterwards in German. I passed the translation easily, but *Nacherzahlung* was the end of my studies.

I visited the instructor, Professor Nikolowsky, but how could I make him understand my difficulties when I didn't understand them myself?

"You just try to put on paper what you hear. Then I'll let you read the story, and after that you can write it down in your own words," Professor Nikolowsky promised.

I sat in the exam, and the instructor read his German story. The sounds were mumbled and muttered in his throat; I couldn't see anything on the lips. I didn't distinguish one single word. I couldn't write anything at all, and the instructor had promised to help only after I got at least something down on paper.

I panicked. I collected my things and fled the lecture room. This was the end. I couldn't continue any more. I wanted to get away from there. But what would I do now?

I walked along the streets without seeing anything. I waded across the street in snow sludge.

"Are you deaf or blind?" The driver's angry voice hit me, coming from the truck standing beside me in the middle of the crossing.

I don't know, I can't think . . . Deaf or blind? At that moment I was both. I was blind to the fact that I was deaf . . .

I had to go somewhere. I went to the cinema. In the dark room it was easier to sink into my own sorrow and let the despair beating inside me hurt so much it almost felt better. Tony Curtis was on the screen, playing the role of a man who succeeds and therefore gets destroyed. The price of success! I, for my part, didn't succeed at all. Do I get destroyed because I don't succeed?

Somewhere in my subconscious, however, there dwelt an idea. I remembered a flyer I had seen on the notice board at the university. "The University Forest Library accepts trainees." After a half-year's practice I could apply to study to become a librarian. The following day I went to see the librarian. Her lips didn't move much, but I did get through the interview. I started work right

— 43 —

away. I marked all arriving mail on cards, arranged the magazines in the reading room, carried returned books to storage and arranged them on the shelves. Finally I felt I was doing something that took me somewhere.

After two months the truth was revealed. It was part of the training to take my turn on duty behind the circulation counter.

"I don't know . . . it's so hard for me to hear the telephone ringing . . . I can't hear the names of the books when the customers ask for something that's not familiar to me. Somehow I just don't distinguish the titles. Maybe I don't know how to concentrate."

It was impossible for me to say that I didn't hear.

Another employee, with whom I had my afternoon tea and who often went and got doughnuts for us, looked at me sympathetically. She didn't tell the librarian anything, but she ran to the telephone for me, and if she noticed that I was having difficulty with a customer, she came to help. Sometimes I told the customer that the book she wanted was out for the moment, which helped. There weren't too many customers, and the telephone rarely rang.

I finished my half year of practice. I applied to the Institute of Social Science to study for a library degree. In the interview, library counselor Helle Kannila asked if I had speech problems (what a considerate word!). It was easy for me to tell her that I "didn't hear too well" and that that had an effect on my speech. If someone else had interviewed me, the door to the university would have stayed closed to me in spite of my good grades. But Helle Kannila was a very open and understanding person; I've met only a few like her in my life.

I got in and studied for the library degree. I got married. Keke was born, I got my degree, I left the university completely. I got a job at the town library in Imatra where my in-laws lived. Jukka was at sea and then at the Kotka Maritime College. Joppe was born. I worked, looked after the children, traveled on Jukka's ships.

I didn't know anything of other hearing-impaired people, nor did I know about the technical aids—flashing doorbells and baby alarms—that could have saved me from sleepless nights and unnecessary tension. My work at the library went well, and my colleagues were nice.

When Jukka started his sea-captain course, the whole family moved to

[handwritten marginalia: other than friends, people much don't help]

Kotka. I had to leave my good position in Imatra. In Kotka I didn't get a new job—the other (hearing) applicant was "better qualified."

When Jukka finished school, became a sea captain and began to specialize in port organization and cargo-handling systems, he told me that it was my turn to finish the studies that I had interrupted eight years earlier.

"Take subjects that don't require hearing and in which you can advance."

The idea seemed impossible. I felt as if I had a big lump in my chest if I even thought about the university building. I hated it tremendously, its columns and stairs, its Greek statues and barren lecture rooms that had roman numerals on them. When I visited the capital and walked past the building, I saw it as an enemy who had humiliated me and ruined my dreams and my self-esteem.

I did go to the library and glance at the examination requirements. I skipped quickly over German philology; it was still a sore spot for me. Gradually I started to feel a strange attraction toward those books that were listed among the examination requirements in education. I knew I had to try.

I had my friend Mari Miettinen with me at the university. I took a completely different path this time. Mari listened for me and wrote down the information I needed, and teachers in the department were flexible.

I wonder if anyone has ever heard of a student who has chosen her major based on the fact that the teachers in that subject are the most flexible communicators at the university? I couldn't even imagine where I would need education, but it became my major.

After the first exam everything started to roll right along. I enjoyed studying. I didn't need to worry if I heard or not, because Mari listened for me, and if she wasn't there, the others helped.

When we lived in Kotka, Riitta Suomela asked me to attend the annual meeting of the Deaf Association in Lappeenranta. I had met Riitta a couple of years earlier, because I saw her interviews in a women's magazine and wrote to her. Finally I had a contact with another hearing-impaired person.

I left for Lappeenranta to go to the meeting. I felt as if I were being drawn along by the current of a stream. When I sat there in the auditorium I felt the interest floating around me: "Who, who? Who is that new person among us?" During the break I met the president of the association, Runo Savisaari. He talked to me with clear mouth movements. Then a young woman approached me whose name was Liisa Kauppinen.

"We have been thinking how we could talk to you," she said slowly and clearly.

I was surprised. It had always been I who figured out how I could talk to others.

After the meeting I happened to meet Ella Mattila, a distinguished elderly lady whom I had seen going into our apartment house. For a year we had lived in the same building on Karhuvuori in Kotka without knowing that we both were deaf.

Ella Mattila led me into the deaf world and taught me my first signs. She took me to the Deaf Club in Kotka and to some events the church arranged for deaf people. Liisa Kauppinen sent the pastor for the deaf, Lauri Paunu, to visit me. He arranged a sign language instructor for me and familiarized me with things that are important to deaf people.

After a couple of years Ella Mattila was elected chairman of the Deaf Association; I was elected secretary. Soon I got elected to the educational committee, after that to other committees, and finally, to the board. All of a sudden a new, richer life began for me.

When I got my bachelor's degree, Jukka admitted, "I didn't quite believe in the beginning that you had the strength to study to the end. But soon I could see that you'd manage well."

There it is now, the white paper with its seal, kept in a safe in the bank—the piece of paper that will never bring me money or status but that is still extremely valuable to me. It is visible proof of something I have accomplished together with Jukka.

However, even after all this, once in a while I am struck by a lack of faith.

Like now, here on the island.

It takes me a couple of months to assure myself that I can teach deaf children. This is in spite of the fact that Clyde, the American, has the same combination of subjects as I do for his degree. In his country deaf people can work as teachers of the deaf. In my country the teacher has to be without any visible disabilities.

"Come to my country," Clyde says. "There deaf people get work according to their education in many fields, even positions of leadership."

No, I don't want to go to America. I want my own country to learn not to waste people's abilities, including those of deaf people.

I say I want to learn more American Sign Language before I begin to teach. I know this is an excuse, because one doesn't learn sign language from books but from talking with deaf people. Sometimes I remember Kenneth making my name sign at Columbus Square, and I know that one day I will start working at the school.

do you agree?
this may be overly optimistic

DO YOU BELONG AMONG US?

I dress in a bright-colored dress, the same one I had on when I visited the school for the deaf on Open Door Day so it might be easier for the children to remember me. I walk to the road. The bus comes right away before anybody gets a chance to offer me a ride. "The bus" is a van with a cover over a frame and narrow benches. I climb up. I am given room on the bench, but I don't know where to put my feet because the floor is full of baskets and bundles.

We fly along the road. I hold tight to the bench. Hair and skirts are flying in the rushing stream of air. Every moment I feel like I'm falling onto the baskets of plantains and yams. Near the marketplace I tap on the frame of the van as a signal. The van stops. I jump out and push my fare through the open window to the driver.

I wonder when I was last in a hurry? Even now I have so much extra time that I can step into the market hall. My favorite seller is sleeping deeply on the bench by the doorway, but the man in the next stall prods him awake when he sees me getting closer—and straightens himself on the same bench, looking satisfied.

I buy a papaya, lettuce, a couple of cucumbers.

"Tomatoes?"

I'm a bit doubtful. Tomatoes look delicious but cost an awful lot. They don't grow well in this climate. Also, my money is gone.

The woman looks for a pen and writes on the paper under the fruit. That's the only paper she has; she counts the prices on her hands.

"I'll give you a pound of tomatoes and you will bring the money the next time." She's got me as a regular customer because of her flexible communication!

good sense
good business

— 48 —

In the park a man is playing a flute, sitting under a tree on a network of roots that spreads high and wide.

There are children already in the schoolyard. Nobody pays any attention to my arrival. I say "Hello" by waving my hand, but I don't get an answer to my greeting. Kenneth is reading comics, one of the boys is jumping on the roof of a low building, two girls are leaning quietly on the fence. Pencils stick out of their thick pigtails.

Behind the iron gate, people standing at the bus stop are staring at the children, their heads visible over the barred fence. I am angry. Are these deaf children foreign creatures whose signing you have to gape at like that?

The children know that they are being stared at. They don't seem to mind, but they avoid signing anyway. The spectators act as if it's a miracle when someone uses his hands to tell another person something. The children from the neighboring school know the tricks. They come and tease Kenneth and Joseph. The boys respond with high-pitched shouts that are as much a wonder to the spectators as the language of hands.

"Go away!" I am really angry, so angry that the boys at the gate pay attention and go away.

Gregory comes and lifts up my hair. He nods. There it is—my hearing aid, under my hair. I don't keep it in my pocket because the rustle of the clothes against the microphone bothers me. Gregory himself has a huge hearing aid hanging from his shirt pocket.

"Do you remember me? We met during the Open Door Day."

I try to sign to Theresa and speak at the same time with clear mouth movements, but Theresa is just smiling her mysterious smile.

"Deaf!" Kenneth points at Theresa. Of course, I know that Theresa is deaf, that's why I'm signing to her as I would sign to a deaf person in Finland, except that I use English and American Sign Language now.

I realize that these children can't read lips because they've never learned worlds that they can read from the lips. To be able to lipread, one has to know the language being spoken. Without that, the lip movements are meaningless.

My spirits sink. I expected a more enthusiastic reception, but the children don't seem to react in any special way to my arrival. And I don't understand their signing at all.

All of a sudden, all the children brighten up, putting one hand in the C-form under the chin. Clyde rides into the yard with his beard and his bag, and I feel right away how unseen strands go from Clyde to every child. The boys circle around Clyde's motorbike.

"This is Raija," Clyde signs. "Do you remember her? She has come to work with us."

The children give me a quick glance, and suddenly the whole crowd is inside pulling down chairs from a pile against the wall. Everybody eventually has a chair to sit on except Gregory, whose chair is falling to pieces. Gregory pulls a chair from under Kenneth; they squabble and fight, and one chair completely splits apart. In the meantime, Clyde has drawn the blackboard full of lines, and somehow we finally reach the point where everybody has an undamaged chair to sit on. Everybody is sitting very still, although I know from experience how big a temptation it is for deaf people to sign all the time because it's so quiet and convenient.

"Today we have news"—news of the day. Today is Monday, it's warm and windy. Joseph has new white shoes. No, they are brown. Clyde is trying out the children's attention and their knowledge of colors.

The boys don't sit still for a moment. I look at Kenneth wonderingly. It is as if there are two boys inside him, the shy and appealing one whom I met at the Square, and now the other one who wants to rule the roost, who knows everything best, and who mocks and teases the others who haven't learned as well as he.

In the middle of everything, Kenneth turns to me and fingerspells. What does he mean? He fingerspells more slowly.

F-A-T-H-E-R.

Does Kenneth want to see if I know the hand alphabet?

No, I know what Kenneth really means.

"Do you speak the same language as we? Do you belong among us?"

I would like him to consider me one of them, I would like to explain that I come from far north where there are many deaf people and that we sign a bit differently than you do down here.

The news is on the board. The notebooks are dealt out and pencils sought. There doesn't seem to be enough for everybody, although the girls have their pencils in their pigtails. The children copy the writing from the board into their notebooks. The desk is small and low, put together out of plywood and rough planks. It's made to fit the small morning children, not these big ones. They have to write in uncomfortable positions on their laps, on chairs, wherever. What a way to learn how to write correctly!

Kenneth finishes first. Now he can't help bothering those who are still scribbling. Poor Gregory has not got past the first line, because he is writing the same letter over and over again.

The notebooks are collected, and Clyde brings in a box. Boys dig out sports gear from it and vanish through the door. I thought that they'd gone out to the sports field, but when I look into the hallway, that's where they are, jumping with both feet together as Clyde counts on his fingers how many times each of them can jump.

I stay with the girls. They go and get their drawing pads. In their notebooks they've drawn houses, but the walls of Filipa's house are all slanting, and Theresa laughs and mocks her.

"Ih!" Filipa pushes her notebook toward me demandingly. Her whole body is saying, "You draw a house for me so that Theresa can't laugh at me, I don't know how to."

Confused, I draw a house. It will be better than Theresa's house, and now it's Filipa's turn to mock. Soon the girls are at each other's hair. I separate them, but Filipa is already going to the door, crying. I bring her back. I pat her shoulder, I try to explain that we are all deaf, we have to be nice to each other and help each other. But of course the girls don't understand what I'm telling them. I don't know how I can express it for them. Explaining demands words and concepts that they don't yet know.

The girls are coloring the house. They like coloring, but don't dare to choose the colors themselves, asking me what color the roof is and what color the door. Oh boy! Somewhere inside them there must be imagination and a need to create, to express themselves. How can I draw that out, or is it too late already?

The boys come in all sweaty, but there's no place for them to get washed. There's a washbasin in the bathroom, but the water has been cut off.

We start to clean up the classroom—the chairs and tables must go back by the walls, the board must be clean. Dust flies when we sweep the rough floor.

Finally we're all perspiring and dirty, and we can't even wash our hands!

Clyde takes pen and paper and writes: "Are you frustrated?"

I am a bit surprised.

"No, I don't have any reason to be frustrated. But shaken, I am for sure."

I am shaken not because the children have so little language base on which to build their education, but because of the fact that the children don't realize that they have similarities among themselves—that they are all deaf. In Finland I've seen what close contact there is among the deaf, but these deaf pupils don't realize that they have each other and have a lot in common.

So many times I've noticed the unseen ties that link Clyde with each child. Clyde even highlights this feeling by using big signs and by fingerspelling with both hands stretched forward toward the children. But the children don't seem to have any ties with each other.

"You will notice that there are both bad days and good days," Clyde writes. "We can't follow an exact schedule. The day's program depends on the feelings of the children and how many of them are at school. We'll keep the school going and make progress as well as we can."

I walk down the hot street into the center of town. Even now, at the coolest season, it's hot in town. I wonder how I will ever move about when the real hot weather arrives.

An air-conditioned hardware store seems like an oasis. I don't have any other shopping to do except to buy a few notebooks for Joppe, but I take my time and cool off, looking at things on the shelves.

Kenneth, Joseph, and Victor are loafing next to the rack of comics. They longingly look through the magazines whose covers show monsters, vampires, iron men, strange creatures from another planet.

"Book, buy!" Kenneth signs.

I can see how much they're drawn to those magazines. I reach for my pocketbook.

"Which one do you want?"

Kenneth points to a magazine showing a vampire with its long fingernails spread, ready to stab its victim.

No, I don't want to give money for this kind of trash.

"No, not that one!"

I take another magazine from the shelf.

"First Kenneth reads, then Kenneth gives to Joseph, then Joseph to Victor, and Victor gives it back to me."

It feels more right that I don't buy the magazine for anybody to own.

I bring the things to the cashier and take my bag from the locker.

". . . teacher?" the man says, giving me my bag. He nods towards the boys.

"Yes," I say, wondering if I can really call myself a teacher. Jukka would say "Yes" without thinking any more about it. Where have I gotten this feeling of inadequacy?

When I give the children their comics, they don't thank me.

"Shouldn't we teach them to say thanks?" I write to Clyde the following day.

"They forget so easily. People spoil them and give them everything when they see that they're deaf. But we can try to teach them to say thank you," Clyde writes back.

Manners are best learned by practice. From now on I demand that the children thank me. I give a notebook or a pencil to Valerie or Joseph or Victor. They take it and turn away at once. But I tap them on the shoulder. When they turn, I move my hand from my mouth and down, forwards: "Thank you." The children repeat the sign. I'd like to teach the children more respect for one another. I'd like to teach them that one should not mock those who learn slowly. I wonder if a picture story could help?

"FA-FA-FA"

"We have news. The weather is sunny, cool, and windy.

"The day is clear. Gregory is late. Today is Thursday. You come to school. We are all fine."

The two hours in school start with news. What day is it, what is the weather like, how are the children, who is in school today, what special things have happened? The news is written on the board, and the children copy it into their notebooks. The language has to be simple, the words familiar, with only one or two new words added every week.

Kenneth remembers almost all the words that have been taught. He wants to show his skill; he signs quickly and vigorously, as if to show how much he knows. There's an expression on his face like that of a distance runner, painfully trying to reach the finish line, wanting to be the best of all. Kenneth's fingers snap fast through the finger alphabet, they bend toward each other as if he wants to highlight the letters. "This is an A, and I know how to do it exactly right."

Joseph knows almost as much as Kenneth, but he behaves more calmly. One can see that he has had a good home and a good childhood. Joseph lives with his grandmother, who visits the school often and brings fruit to Clyde.

"Who is here?" Clyde asks.

Kenneth's fingers are already swift as lightning with the answer.

"Kenneth is here. I am here."

"Joseph is here. I am here," Joseph answers calmly and precisely.

"Gregory?" Clyde looks at Gregory, who has come to school late as usual, with a packet of sticky coconut candy in his pocket of the kind that women sell on the corner. It's not actually any news that Gregory is late.

But Gregory is absent-minded; he doesn't have the energy to concentrate on learning. He lives in his own world, which he only rarely leaves. I've practiced writing with him, but it seems as if there are three of us at the table. Gregory's friend is there, an unseen comrade whom Gregory talks to. In a while, Gregory returns to reality to write his letters, which never seem to get finished. He wants them to be perfect. He writes until the paper is worn through if I'm not there to tell him, "That's good, it's good," and even mark with a red pen *Good*.

"Who is here?" Clyde repeats and signs as a model: "Gregory is here. I am here." But in reality Gregory is not here. He is far away in his own land.

Victor signs to Kenneth, laughs, grins, is having fun. Clyde taps him, and Victor verifies without any trouble: "Victor is here. I am here," and goes on with his playing.

"Theresa is here. I am here," Theresa signs with a bit of uncertainty. She knows the signs well. Her vocabulary is not quite as large as Kenneth's or Joseph's, and she doesn't have Kenneth's self-confidence. But she has been in school almost every afternoon for two years and has acquired the facts that have been so patiently taught. Theresa lives with her mother and four sisters; I've met them in town. I can tell that the girls have a good relationship.

Filipa is next. "Am I fine?" "No, am I here?" Filipa corrects herself. She signs fast and assuredly, but she doesn't understand the meanings of the words. She only repeats mechanically what she remembers. Already, even this early, Filipa has been left behind. She is in the slow group.

The same is true for Valerie. But now, Valerie signs correctly, "Valerie is here. I am here." Valerie sometimes knows the lesson perfectly well, but she doesn't care about learning. All learning for her is "bad." She just wants to color coloring books all day long.

I teach Valerie and Filipa in the afternoon while Clyde is teaching his clever group: Kenneth, Joseph, Theresa, and Victor. I've been able to cut down the coloring time, but I haven't really made much progress. Day after day I teach the words "boy" and "girl," and I don't know if the girls understand or remember even these simple words. Clyde has advised me to make sure that, by signing, speaking, writing, fingerspelling, and any other possible means, I get the girls to understand each new word. Filipa writes "Flipopo" when she should write

crocosm — typical group

— 55 —

good point

"Filipa Popo." Valerie writes her name "Valerei." She doesn't remember her last name.

Andrew is not in school today. And if he were, he would wander around the room, and Clyde would let him wander. Andrew is rarely in school, and when he is, the best he can do is just be with us and experience what little he can. It's better than nothing. Getting away from home into another environment can mean something; learning even one or two words can mean something, and learning five signs can mean having contact with other deaf people.

The children have their own signs, which they used before they started school, and they have the signs that they invent spontaneously to describe a thing or a condition. But it's difficult to know what the other person means, exactly. Common signs that mean the same thing to all the children are better, but some words have different shades of meaning for each child, depending on personal experiences.

A girl is a girl, a house a house, that's clear; but the word "mother" can have different meanings. For Kenneth it means a woman who gives him food and washes his clothes. Many deaf children live with some relative who has taken the child in, who is better able to understand and take care of a deaf child. The child's own mother may be unable to do that, and often has other children to look after.

In the beginning I don't understand anything of the children's signing. I don't know which are from the American Sign Language Clyde has taught them, which are their own signs, and which is just typical lively Latin American gesturing.

One day we're standing in the yard waiting for Clyde to arrive. There are spectators behind the fence, as usual. Andrew has appeared at school again. He has a hearing aid, like Gregory, but the sounds the hearing aid transmits are painful to him. When the other children are shouting, he takes the hearing aid off. Andrew seems like a nice boy, but whenever he's in school there are fights and disturbances.

"Your home?" I sign to Andrew, looking puzzled.

Fa-fa-fa: Andrew's lips form *F* and long *A*, and his hand is waving toward the mountains.

how they understand the words

Samantha's home? Samantha is in the small children's class in the morning and often waits for Andrew to go with her by bus to the village of Fond Assau.

Andrew points with his finger at a house, a roof top. Then with the other hand two sharp roof tops and a stop—there's Samantha's home.

So two roofs away from Andrew's home is Samantha's home. But there are many, many roofs between us and the school—the school is *fa-fa-fa*, and a land beyond the sea is *fa-fa-fa*—as far as the hand can be reached out, and then a sign of an airplane on top of the hand. The thumb, forefinger, and little finger cut the air like the wings of an airplane.

Fa-fa is a sign one of the children has invented and the other children have adopted so strongly that there's no point in explaining to them what the American sign for "far" is like.

Many signs that Clyde teaches change in the children's language into easier ones, like *what* and *who*. It's hard to remember the difference between the words *what* and *who*. And why do the sign in such a complicated manner? So *what* and *who* are signed in the children's sign language just by touching the lips with the forefinger.

I am starting to grasp the children's sign language better. It's like a puzzle—the more pieces you fit into their places, the easier it is to understand. I notice that children use only a few signs in their conversation, but with the help of pantomime they tell little incidents to each other. Their most common communication, however, is squabbling.

The children are constantly shouting, producing their own sounds—high-pitched, piercing, sometimes painful sounds that hurt the ears. The high pitch often kills my hearing aid, like the whistle of the teakettle at home. I don't hear its sound, but all of a sudden when all the different sounds that are transmitted through my hearing aid stop, I know to go and turn off the gas. Sometimes, like Andrew, I turn off my hearing aid. It doesn't help me understand speech, but it helps me notice that there is some sound somewhere, and it covers the constant humming in my ears.

"Papapapapaa." The lips are moving, as in real speech. One could imagine that the children are really speaking, if one didn't know that they have no words with which to speak.

After the two hours have passed in school, after the floor has been swept, the windows closed, the boards washed, after I've sat in the bus and waited for it to leave, looking at the life on Jeremie Street, I ride home. When I arrive, I'm completely exhausted.

I notice that there are bad days and good days. The bad days are not the children's fault. It's not their fault that the important years when language is learned have been wasted for them. No one in their childhood environment has used sign language.

Around a hearing child, there are always words and sounds. They stream in through the ears, into the consciousness. Little by little, the child will learn words and sentences, aping speech and automatically acquiring language.

The deaf child doesn't hear what's going on. He or she might hear sounds but can't distinguish words. The child doesn't learn the language that's being spoken and never starts speaking it. The only possibility for a deaf child to learn the language is by using the eyes. To learn with one's eyes a language whose sounds one should be hearing is an impossible task for a deaf child.

However, the deaf person has to communicate somehow, and that's why the deaf instinctively fall back on sign language. In Finland it has begun to be understood that sign language is the natural language for the deaf to use to make contact with other deaf people, get information and concepts, acquire a circle of friends and broader communication abilities, and take advantage of their opportunities in life.

Here on the island of St. Lucia people don't even understand yet that deaf children are able to learn and that you can talk with them in sign language, although general openness and caring does help the child's life and adjustment.

My starting point was better than these children have had: I heard well enough during those early years when the mother tongue is learned. However, speaking, maintaining clear speech, has been my biggest worry recently, sometimes an even more difficult matter for me than the fact that I don't hear.

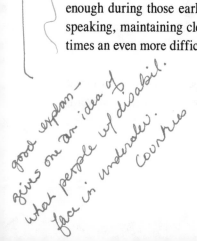

good explan. — gives one an idea of what people w/ disabil. face in underdev. countries

BUT CHILDREN
SHOULD SPEAK!

We have had many good days, and I'm happy. I have sensible work that I feel I can manage. I do, however, have to learn to teach, and I try to keep learning the sign language of the children so I can perform better.

Joy and happiness never last more than a few moments or a day at a time.

"Tomorrow we'll have a visitor from Canada," Clyde tells us one day, all excited. "A lady will come who can find money for us. We'll throw away these miserable chairs and tables and we'll buy new ones. We'll get books and pencils and everything we need."

Clyde has met somebody in Barbados who in turn knows some influential person in Canada who is in the Rotary Club. Now this Canadian organization will send an expert to see if we need help and what kind of help we need.

"What are we going to show the guest tomorrow? Shouldn't we plan ahead a bit?" I ask Clyde.

"No, we should be what we usually are. We can't be hypocritical. A normal day, so that the guest can see that we work in difficult conditions."

The next day Clyde is late. He has been out to lunch with the woman guest and other important people. He arrives looking harried—late, angry, and disappointed.

I can only imagine what has happened: Clyde eating his lunch, forgotten, an outsider. He knows that the subject under discussion is the school whose problems are so important to him, but he is not being asked anything, and he can't tell them anything because nobody seems to be willing to talk with him by writing or signing. He doesn't find out what the others are saying. By the time he

Clyde excluded by group - like admin: fear of deaf schools

arrives at school he is almost bursting—first from wanting to tell and then from rage.

How well I know those situations! In my country people talk and decide things without even asking what the people concerned think of the matter. One has to yell loud before one is noticed. For deaf people to be heard, they have to have the knowledge and the means to express themselves. The deaf must first be able to go to school and learn how their society works. Only after that are they able to express their views and advocate their own programs.

The woman guest arrives. Clyde begins with the news. The children are all quiet, but they're not at their best, because they sense that Clyde is not himself. After the news has been written, the guest wants to tell the children something. She is signing Canadian sign language and speaking at the same time—too many words and concepts that are unfamiliar to the children. I can see that they are sitting stiffly, and there's a curtain between them and the lady; there is no contact.

We form into groups. I have prepared the lesson for the slower group. I attach a picture to the wall. "This is Tom." Today I'll teach the words "to ride." Tom is riding a bicycle in the picture.

At a glance I see how the lady takes Kenneth away and leads him all over the classroom, examines him and tries to find out what he knows. I know that Kenneth knows a whole lot, considering that he started school at the age of 11, is in his third year of school, and has been made to study for two hours every afternoon. But the lady either doesn't know the facts or doesn't understand. She is terrified!

She thinks of all the things a 13-year-old deaf child in her own country already knows. That is not as much as a 13-year-old hearing pupil knows, but it's a lot more than Kenneth knows. Suppose the lady had chosen Filipa or Valerie, she might have fainted from fright!

Kenneth knows that the lady is not satisfied with him, and looks troubled. He knows everything that has been taught; what does this lady want from him?

". . . on the contrary, I think that these children first of all should have been taught to speak and to understand speech from the lips. I don't accept signing, and you only teach by signing."

Clyde tries to explain, but the lady is like a wall. Now *she* is the one who is *this visitor "doubly foreign"*

visitor — too quick to judge

deaf, deaf to the facts. I stand by quietly, although I should have explained to the lady what the truth is.

Dear lady, after a two-day visit you don't know anything about this island. And when you don't know this country, how can you say anything about its concerns, no matter how much of an expert you are? Work in our school for at least a month. Maybe after that you'll start understanding these children. Listen to what Clyde and I have to say, because we're experts, too. Some matters we know better than a hearing person can ever know. Can't you understand that speaking is not the same as knowing a language? The best that we can give these children is a common language with which they can communicate with each other, so that they'll at least have somebody who will understand when they explain their experiences and feelings. They will never be able to do that in spoken English.

They have to learn to communicate with each other, at least to start with, and this is so awfully important and you can't understand it, and perhaps you never will.

But nothing comes out of my mouth.

The following day the lady is gone, stupefied, with information about our backward teaching. Our pupils don't speak nor understand speech from the lips, you know! Poor Clyde! We have to go on using the same falling-apart chairs and falling-down blackboards!

We all are frustrated, Clyde and me and especially Kenneth. From the beginning he is restless, so that he has to be removed from the class. But he keeps disturbing our teaching from outdoors, keeps hitting things outside, and throwing rocks. The day will be a bad one.

theft of money

At the marketplace when I want to buy vegetables I notice that my purse is empty. All my strength drains away, because I know for sure that I had three dollars in my purse when I left home. Someone among the children must have visited my bag. It's always in the office, the office door is open, the children go in there to sharpen their pencils, and Gregory is always searching for something.

It's all my fault. I should have kept my eye on the bag. But my heart is heavy. I wish that the bus would leave; it's completely full already. But no, the driver is greedy for more and more passengers. The children in their school uniforms are sitting on each other's laps; beside the driver there is a pile of fruit baskets. Now another box is forced inside. Finally we start our journey, lunging for-

cultural (etc) probs — they to help + they steal!

ward. More passengers are taken in from the bus stops. The bus is like Mary Poppins's bag: although it's full, there's always room for some more. Sweat runs down my body, and it's difficult to breathe.

I decide to start walking home from school. Three miles—it will work if it's not too hot.

AMONG US GIRLS

exploring differences

outsiders' view of these girls = (?)

The girls are interested in me, and I grow closer to them. They wonder about my light skin, which Kenneth calls yellow. Theresa signs "red," the letter R brushing her lips. She sees that I wear lipstick. Filipa moves her thumb against the other fingers.

"How much does lipstick cost?" she wants to know. She's interested in make-up and tells me that she once put make-up on her eyes at her friend's house. She wonders how much eye shadow and mascara cost.

The girls are pulling their hair straight from the roots, questioningly, but then Filipa bursts out laughing. She notices that my hair is naturally straight; I don't need to straighten it. On the contrary, I go to the hairdresser to put curls in, not to straighten my hair. But how handy their curly hair is in this climate. The wind doesn't mess it up, nor does it get wet and go flat in this hot, moist climate.

Theresa looks wonderingly at the birthmarks I have on my face and arms. What are they? Theresa is a beautiful, proud-looking girl, pure-featured and velvet-skinned. Now I know the reason for her shy smile, which doesn't show her teeth at all. Theresa has big holes in her two front teeth. Soon there will be only the stumps left.

During the handicraft lessons we sit at the table and try to sew, but Filipa's hands have a hard time staying with the handiwork; they are explaining the whole time how she likes babies, she wants many, many babies. She wants to walk with her big stomach out and be envied by all the girls, and then walk with a beautifully dressed baby in her arms. The baby's dress is white, and she has a white knitted bonnet on her head. Filipa signs that she already has a boyfriend. Maybe her stomach really will get round one of these days.

Valerie shows with burning eyes how she wants to get married. Her veil is long and white, she will get married in the church, and then she will buy a car and a house and fly "fa-fa-fa." And there will be six babies. Poor Valerie, on this island the deaf are not allowed to get married, the law says so . . . In Finland that kind of law was repealed.

Theresa is snorting. She is a clever girl and doesn't like Filipa's and Valerie's constant babbling. But then Filipa and Valerie start squabbling that Theresa already has a baby.

"No, no," Theresa presses her thumb against her forefinger and middle finger, frightened.

I nod, calming her. Of course not. Theresa doesn't have a baby. Let the girls squabble as they wish. Let's do handicrafts.

I have to watch what the girls are doing all the time. The thread should be passed beautifully through the fabric, but the stitches don't seem to become regular. Filipa has the habit of doing everything too fast; she doesn't stop to wait for advice. During the math lesson she has time to scribble through her whole notebook while I teach the first page to Valerie.

Filipa doesn't need advice because she thinks she knows everything. She knows how to write letters and numbers. It's hard to explain to her that although her letters look right, they don't form any sensible words.

Once in a while, the girls dance. Even without music they sense the right rhythm. They want to be like other girls; they want to dance, wear make-up, go walking with a boyfriend.

I start laughing when Filipa shows how boys stare at her when she goes by and how she looks back, fluttering her eyelashes, and what will happen after that. Filipa enters into the spirit of her pantomime; she is no longer in the classroom, but on the street where all this has taken place.

"Sick." Valerie indicates her throat with her middle finger. I tell her to open up her mouth wide. I can see all her rotten black teeth and behind them the red, swollen throat. I look for the aspirin in my purse.

Valerie looks happy. I take all her aches seriously because I understand that she wants attention and sympathy. The girl's aching teeth and her constantly inflamed throat won't get better with just sympathy, but it does bring some relief.

Theresa had a sore throat as well. The nurse has visited and has given the children shots. Filipa tells me how she stood in a queue, then pulled her sleeve up *isolation even stronger for deaf in foreign country*

and got a shot. I tell the girls how Keke and Joppe got shots when they were babies, so that they wouldn't catch infectious diseases.

I get a doll from the cabinet. Now we're at the children's clinic. Joppe is lying on my lap; he is just a little baby. The nurse gives the shot, Joppe's mouth widens, but he doesn't cry. Then another shot, and Joppe doesn't cry this time, either. I sign, fling my hands around, gesticulate, and all of a sudden I notice that Clyde is passing by. He laughs. The girls around the table look happy and smiling. I have "spoken" the same language as they, not a stiff language learned from dictionaries. From that time on Clyde signs to me more and more, and we use paper and pencil less and less.

And still I can't fill the empty space in Clyde's life on the island, where he's far away from his family and friends. There are no deaf adults here with whom he can chat easily.

There must be deaf adults on the island, but where are they? Clyde rides a lot on his motorbike around the island. This bearded American teacher of the deaf, the one with the rucksack, is known on the island. From his sack he digs out paper and pen and one can "talk" with him—unless one only knows patois, the local language that can't be written at all.

Clyde searches for deaf people on his trips to the fishing villages or to the houses and villages in the mountains and the banana valleys. Thus far he has met only six deaf adults. One of them is George, the man who sells newspapers in town.

I have been on the island for half a year and I don't know any other deaf adults besides George and one slightly crazy woman. She walks past our house, hips swaying, a big box or bucket on top of her head. She notices me when I stand on the other side of the road at the bus stop. She crosses the road, looks first to the right and then to the left with a stiff neck, holding on to the box. She gestures as much as she can with that swaying burden on her head. At least she can roll her eyes, and that she does, flattering and appealing. Now she takes my hand, touches all the five fingers and finally draws a circle on my palm, stretches out a begging hand, pats my cheek. She knows that I am nice and will give her fifty cents because—she taps on her stomach—she is hungry.

I'm surprised. I haven't seen this woman before. I try to think where she could live, if she is completely deaf or just pretending deafness to get money.

The woman is standing in front of me with her hand stretched out; she smiles flirtatiously with her toothless mouth.

But I don't have fifty cents for her. I need my coins for bus fare, because I'm on my way to town.

But the woman doesn't believe me. Of course I have money; I am white, am I not? Maybe American. I dig ten cents from my purse, No, it is not good enough, the woman gestures again. All the fingers of one hand and a zero on the palm, and patting me on the cheek. Finally when she believes that I really won't give her more, she thanks me, pats my cheek, sways herself along with her box in the direction she was going. I stay and watch her move toward the curve in the road.

Another time the woman comes to our yard with her drooping crocheted lace hat, shows her stomach, and flirts again, but she doesn't reach out to pat my cheek because I'm standing on the balcony. I laugh; her gestural language is in its way quite talented. But I won't give her money, because if I did she would come again and again, and I wouldn't get any peace.

But what if, instead, there were old clothes! The woman tries again. She lifts her skirt hem and shows her worn petticoat. I lift my own skirt and show her that I don't have a petticoat at all, and Zenia laughs by her washing pail.

"I will come back at four o'clock and then you will give me money and food," the woman gestures.

She takes her bucket, throws me a kiss, and walks with her swaying stride through the garden to the road.

The woman does not come back at four, nor do I see her for a long time. I would like to know more about her and other deaf adults—where do they live, how do they live, what is their sign language like? But here on the island you can't hurry too much. You have to wait until things come your way. 🐦

ADJUSTING TO THE ISLAND WAY OF LIFE

The island and its climate wake a person up to a new life and give a new, more relaxed feeling, but at the same time they subtract something from your former energy.

I always experience Nature very strongly—the sun and warmth of the island, which now is becoming heat and sweat, but especially this unique atmosphere. After you've lived here for a while you start to see and experience something else besides its exotic, paradisiacal features.

Sometimes I feel I'm up to my ears in it all. At the marketplace and on Jeremie Street I see only dirt and misery: decayed shacks, dirty, weatherbeaten feet, the torn clothes that people wear, drunkards on the streets, open drains that slowly flow by the barrack-style rental accommodations, drains into which the inhabitants constantly throw new waste. Tin cans, bottles, plastic, mud, waste, secretions, smells in the hot standing air. Poverty, jealousy, hatred. I miss my home country and everything that is unique and good there, but still I wouldn't like to leave the island yet. Soon again I begin to experience life over here as colorful and challenging and inspiring.

Often I have a bad conscience because the boys don't seem to enjoy life on St. Lucia. They don't tell me about their troubles the way they used to; they're not little boys any more. But I notice that they don't get very interested in anything, and I guess the island isn't a rich environment for European youth at that stage of development. Sometimes I feel that the boys just are more realistic than I am.

On the other hand, my own experiences depend so much on what I see, and the visual offerings over here are quite royal. Otherwise my life revolves around the school for the deaf and deaf children.

The boys for their part necessarily experience the cultural differences more strongly. Their words and behavior are easily misunderstood. One local teacher sends Keke out of the classroom because of his "Finnish arrogance"—whatever that means.

All in all, there's nothing miraculous about the island in Keke's and Joppe's opinion, nothing that would compare with peers and hobbies in Finland.

I could do so many things, but days just fly by, and time doesn't mean the same as it does back home. I already live by island time; I am not in a hurry to be anywhere: small tasks, going to the store, a couple of hours at school, fixing dinner, talking with Jukka in the evenings on the balcony. For him, time over here is the same as back home; there's always too little of it, and work has to be bulldozed along at full force.

In the afternoons after lunch I leave for town. It's like driving into a hot furnace. Two hours at school are enough, I could hardly bear any more. When I return home the streets are glowing with heat, and the small buses are crammed full of passengers.

When everybody has come home, we go to the beach. The setting sun is hanging like a big ball close to the horizon. The sand is cool under our feet; it feels wonderful to move vigorously along the beach, to walk or to run in the sand over the waves lazily rolling onto the shore. Small crabs are twirling, frightened, into their holes, which are as straight-walled as if they were made by a drill.

Late in the afternoon our house is full of life. The neighbor's dogs are running around on the balcony. One of them, black-and-white Mickey, guards our house at night. Sometimes at night the wind whizzing through the glass espalier wakes me up. The curtains are swaying. When I look outside, Mickey is sleeping on the balcony chair, and an old boxer snores on the doormat.

Keke's classmate John Eugene comes straight from school to our house and stays for dinner almost every day. The leftovers from dinner I scrape into bowls and take to the dogs. Zenia and Anderson each carries a bag home: eggs, rolls, cheese, chicken legs, and sometimes canned milk for Zenia's children.

Zenia's salary is small, and we can't pay her more than what is common on the island. She lives in a cramped rental room on the slope of the Morne. Her clothes are kept in a suitcase, and she cooks meals outside on a coal pot. The small houses, gray from the rain, sit side by side, everybody knows everybody's business—quarrels, fights, hunger, illnesses, drinking. The area is thick with rum stores, and rum is cheap.

But in this community they also care for each other. Somebody looks after Zenia's children, somebody gives her food if she doesn't have any. Zenia herself gives food to others when she has anything from which to give.

Maybe we could only understand the life on St. Lucia if we lived among these people. Though we are not isolated in some special place for white people, the gap in living standards can still be seen.

The evenings are quiet. Outside the house is wet, soft, warm darkness. Only the light of the lighthouse and the sparkling of fireflies cut the dark. The neighbor girls, Alison and Debbie, are dancing on their balcony. At the other neighbor's house, the maid is still washing dishes; she has much longer days than Zenia. The plane going to Barbados or Martinique rumbles over the house.

We sit on the balcony after dinner, and Jukka tells us what has happened at the port and in the administration buildings, what people have said or done, and why they've acted like this or like that, in Jukka's opinion. Without these sessions I would know much less of the life in St. Lucia.

Sometimes a headlight beam appears on the road. Usually the cars drive up the hill, but sometimes a car turns into the driveway leading to our yard.

Often the visitor is Cornell Charles. He comes up the stairs and sinks with a supple motion onto the balcony couch. He is so tall that I have to crane my neck to see his face.

Cornell is a member of the Port Council, president of the Chamber of Commerce and managing director of the biggest company in St. Lucia, J. Q. Charles.

Cornell helps Jukka understand the behavior and language of the local people. He interprets for Jukka what is behind people's behavior, what they think of things, what caused this event or that reaction. Cornell also describes the political atmosphere and the changes that occur in the political situation on the island.

Cornell's interpretations help Jukka in his decision making. Cornell also is a good balance to Jukka's nature: Jukka may bang his fist on the table in the Port Office and rattle off what he thinks of the matter. That's why, at the port, they started calling Jukka "Moses." Cornell calms him down, tells Jukka not to be so demanding. But Jukka is impatient to get the system working.

And it does work, although sometimes it's difficult to keep things going. Maybe they see at the port that Jukka is not saving himself, either. Even on Sundays he goes to the port to see how the loading of bananas is going. He wants to make sure that everything functions, that everything is in its place.

In spite of that, John Hailwood, the manager of the Geest Banana Company, sometimes phones Jukka and scolds the whole port. He thinks that it doesn't function properly.

Jukka has figured again how the loading capacity of the port could even be better than in Finland. But every day it rains at least a little, and you can't load during rain showers. Banana production is the main livelihood of the island, and it's a trade that demands a lot of attention. From the moment a banana cluster is cut at the banana fields of Cul-De-Sac or Roseau Valley, there is a certain time span in which to get the bananas to the customers in England or elsewhere in Europe. If the banana ship is late, it's a sad story for the Geest Company, the port, and St. Lucia.

But aside from these worries and problems, John Hailwood is our good friend. He lives by the sea in a beautiful white building that I always admire as I wait for the bus. John sends his driver to bring books and National Geographic magazines to the boys, and he invites us for dinner at his home.

We're starting to get a group of good friends on the island. We experience their generosity in many ways, and I worry only about the fact that I can hardly talk with them.

A BOY FROM THE
FISHING SHORE

In the fishing port there is a row of narrow, colorfully painted boats that have been scooped out of big tree trunks. Some of them have a mast and a simple sail, some have a big outboard motor. These unstable boats leave in the mornings for the open sea to fish, with the words "God Protects" painted on the bow, and two or three men, on their way back in the dark night, have a big kingfish as their catch. If they have not had luck fishing, there are only flying fish lying on the bottom of the boat.

The streaks of sunlight grow thinner on the skyline. Men are sitting on boxes playing dominoes. Cartons sitting in the mud on the shore are full of mangoes and oranges that will be loaded onto the boats the following morning. The fruit is taken to Barbados, a flat, almost treeless island.

In the the alleys of the slums, dogs are barking, and chickens lurch back and forth. The little tots with nothing on but a shirt are romping. Smoke rises from the barrels at the square; I've never found out what is smoldering in those barrels. Over the mud there's a plank bridge leading to a small saloon. A dim lamp hangs from the ceiling, swaying; men sit hunched at the bar. Next to the saloon there's a shoemaker's stall; one wall is open and the shoemaker is hammering shoes almost out on the street. Under a mango tree a barber wields his scissors, swiftly, as late as he can still see. (My hairdresser, who now has a fine salon in the center of town, started the same way—a chair under a mango tree, with scissors, a comb and a razor blade for tools.) There are always women in the alleyways who mutter, quarrel, and brandish their fists.

We stand in the fishing port, Jukka and I. We have a lot to watch. We're in a crowd that is waiting for the return of the boats and fish for dinner. Kingfish is especially good; Zenia puts a lot of onion, curry, and tomato in it and fries it in coconut oil. The flying fish are the islanders' "Baltic herring."

Once I watched big sharks being dragged out of the hold, one after another across the bloody deck. A one-eyed captain watched over the operation. (I felt as if I were in the middle of a novel, but it was true.) Keke and Joppe have seen small sharks and barracudas even in offshore waters, but swimming on the island is safe. Big killers don't come close to shore.

In the beginning the islanders didn't want to sell fish to us. The fishermen think that white people have money to buy more expensive food. Fish is scarce and is one of the most important protein sources for the islanders. There's plenty of it in the sea, but the boats and catching equipment are primitive, and neither storage nor selling has been organized very well. Inland, the children often have swollen stomachs, because families there eat mainly bananas in different forms.

Now the fishermen know us. We work and live here. Jukka has a dollar with him. It buys four flying fish, the fisherman says.

"One should get six," Jukka says, and he gets six fish. The wife of the fisherman even cleans them and scatters salt on them. The fishermen stretch out their hands, passing the fish straight from the boats to the customers without any wrapping. If we want the fish wrapped in paper, it has to be bought separately for a couple of cents a sheet from a little boy or from the old woman who is crouched near the boats.

"There's that deaf boy I've been telling you about," Jukka says one evening. "Where?"

I lean toward the group of people and see the boy. He's standing there waiting for someone to buy a piece of paper from the pile he has in his arms—clean, smooth, brown sack paper.

Something about the boy makes an impression. He is standing in the crowd of people and yet is as alone as if he doesn't belong anywhere. His heavy eyelids are curtains over his eyes. He has drawn a shade over himself and hopes nobody ever tries to see what's behind it—that nobody asks him anything, because he wouldn't understand and couldn't answer, and only discomfort would come of it. He must be on guard all the time.

And yet the boy doesn't look humble. His head is proudly and self-consciously erect. Maybe it's just this position of his head and its royal posture that attracted my attention . . . the straight nose is self-assertive. The boy has Indian features.

I push my way through to him. I put my hands over my ears.

"You deaf?"

The boy nods.

"Me also deaf."

A quick look from under the eyelids, and again the curtains drop down.

"You know to write?"

A head shake.

"Your name?"

Head shake. Of course he can't know the American sign for "name." How can I explain to him that I would like to know his name? It appears to me that perhaps he doesn't know that people have names, doesn't know even that he has a name, because perhaps he has never been called by a name. From somewhere I remember the name Alfonso. He can be called Alfonso until I get to know more about him.

"I teach at school."

I show him where the school is. There, behind the park.

Head shake.

The boy shakes his head for almost everything I want to sign to him. We don't have a common language. I can't use the finger alphabet, because he doesn't know any letters, and he doesn't know signs from American Sign Language. I just have to try to find gestures that he'll understand, and even that is difficult, because the whole time he shelters himself, averting his head and hiding behind his concealing eyelids.

"Your home?" I show him sleeping and eating. The boy brightens and swings his hand in a wide circle toward the mountains.

Soon I notice that it has become dark. Lights have been lit on the mountainsides; the lights from the big ships in the bay reflect on the water.

I pantomime washing clothes, stirring food.

"Who washes your clothes, who cooks your meals? Your mother?"

I look at his shirt. It's clean, but torn. His pants have been patched and the legs are cut off under the knee. There's a black band around his ankle. He is barefoot.

The boy points at the sky. I notice, as if awakening, that hundreds of stars have been lit in the dark sky.

Stars and darkness, lights that climb up the mountainsides and reflect on the water. I seem to be experiencing something supraterrestrial. Somewhere on the other side of the stars are the boy's mother and father. And here on the pier of the fishing port is this thin boy in his torn clothes who keeps his forefinger up and nods at the same time as if to assure me of something.

"Me. Alone."

"You wash your clothes and cook your meals?"

"Me. Alone . . . me. Alone."

I go through the crowd to Jukka. I haven't noticed how the crowd has grown and that everyone has been curiously looking at how I've talked with the boy who can't talk.

"Let's give the boy some money. Today there was so little fish on sale that the boy didn't get his paper sold."

"It's better if we buy him bread." I go back to the boy. I tell him to follow. The boy comes without question into the car.

We drive through dim streets to the bakery. Inside Jukka points at two sixty-cent breads. The baker puts them into a bag, and the boy is left standing in the street with a brown bag under his arm, with the twisty tops of the bread sticking out of it.

"I come to fish market. Me your friend." I gesture to the boy before I climb into the car.

But then we decide that we will take the boy to his home and see where he actually lives. We drive over the bridge, past the police station and the Pepsi-Cola bottling plant. The road winds abruptly to the Mountain Morne. We climb even higher—the boy swings his hand—still farther up, until we stop.

The boy steps out of the car at a spot where no houses can be seen. Behind the red clay ditch there's a hole in a row of trees. The boy vanishes through the hole into the darkness.

We sit still in the car, pondering.

"Let's go and see what's there," Jukka says rapidly.

We climb over the sharp edge of the ditch; the red clay is slippery. There's a steep slope down to the valley in front of us. From somewhere comes a dim shimmer of light. Afterwards I don't remember if there was moonlight or if the light was reflected from the town or from the houses on the slope above.

We see the slightly shining tops of palms and banana trees. Above them are lemon trees and mango trees. Behind those, a dark house gleams in reflected light; we can't distinguish it clearly, but we wait for the boy to go inside and turn the lights on.

But the lights aren't lit. The boy didn't go into that house; he has disappeared into the darkness. I can see with my imagination that he goes into a hovel. There's a pile of rags in the corner, the boy bends over them, cuts the bread and falls asleep. Suppose it rains during the night. . .?

GOOD DAYS AND
BAD DAYS

why does Miss Johnson help?

The school functions mostly on a volunteer basis. Once in a while Miss Johnson comes to help. She teaches Gregory or replaces Clyde when he is away. I don't know why she comes, because she doesn't seem to have any interest in deaf children and their problems or in teaching them. She is angry and irritated at the children and laughs at their "stupidity" or "peculiarities."

I don't join her in laughing. I take seriously what the children say, and try to think what they really mean. The children's gestures, facial expressions, signs, behavior, all show something of their thoughts, feelings, and hopes. And one has to find something good resulting from one's work. There's no reason to laugh at the children. It's better to praise what you can praise than to put down a child who hasn't had a chance to learn much yet.

When Clyde goes to Barbados for a few days, Miss Johnson will come to school to help me take care of the teaching.

We gather the children around the table and tell them that we'll now draw the flowers, trees, and fruits of the island. I show them pictures because I know that they can't get started without models.

To my surprise something has happened to Filipa. She draws her paper full of balloons, blue, red, green, all colors. Miss Johnson says that balloons don't mean anything; they're not flowers or fruit. But that's not important. The most important thing is that Filipa has learned to express herself in colors!

I show the children pictures of papaya, hibiscus, flamboyant. I don't know how it all starts. Kenneth is yelling in high-pitched, piercing shrieks that make Miss Johnson's face grim. That's Kenneth's intention; he wants her life to be unbearable. He yells like a factory whistle, and all the while he teases Theresa.

Finally Theresa can't take it any more, and hits back. The chairs and the plywood walls in between fall down. Crayons fly into the air. Suddenly Kenneth has scissors in his hand; he threatens to pierce Theresa's eyes with them. Nobody can take the scissors away. Kenneth has a fierce look in his eyes. He's like a wild animal in a cage.

Kenneth goes and gets the hammer and starts breaking a table. Bang, bang, bang. I do something I've never done before, twist the boy's arm behind his back to try to get the scissors away from him, but he has the speed and strength of an enraged being. I can't do anything.

I suddenly realize that the other children have been sitting still the whole time, staring at Kenneth. Andrew's hearing aid knob is hanging on his shirt front. Kenneth's cries have been too much for him, too. Gregory's aid is in its place, and he is far away, as usual. There's wonder in the children's eyes. And yet they know Kenneth, know his desire to tease, his direct, constant mockery toward those who are not as clever as he is.

Theresa is crying. I shiver from anger, fear, and lack of strength. The whole incident has been a surprise. I had guessed that Kenneth has this side to him, but what I didn't know was how strongly his frustration can come out. Talented deaf people get frustrated more easily. They know that they would be able to learn, to go far, but their impairment is an obstacle. Kenneth feels it instinctively.

But right at this moment, when Kenneth is standing with the scissors in his hand and a fierce look in his eyes, I don't have one single, sympathetic thought in my mind, no pity, nothing. Kenneth's rage is not directed toward me, but toward Miss Johnson, for whom Kenneth was as invisible as air. Or do we both, to Kenneth, represent the mother who has rejected him, left him without love?

The next day I go to school with mixed feelings. I've thought about the crisis all evening long, but I can't find any other solution except to hide all scissors and tools. I have asked Jukka for advice. He hasn't quite understood how two women can't get a half-grown boy thrown out or sent home. I am wondering the same thing. But the day goes well; Kenneth is peaceful. The next day is also good, and the following day I decide not to hide the scissors any more.

We have a health day and talk about health care, washing, brushing teeth, and other important matters. Jukka has given all the children toothbrushes. We deal them out and practice brushing teeth. We have to do something for the children's teeth. Every time I see Theresa's, Victor's, or Valerie's front teeth with big, black, wide-open holes in them, I ponder how that damage could be repaired. We tell the children that the dentist can fill the holes, and then the teeth will be beautiful and won't ache.

Theresa touches her eyes, puts her hand to her forehead, and opens her arms.

"I have not seen a dentist and I don't know where he is." She is interested.

"Write note to mother, where dentist," she gestures.

I am doubtful. If I send a note home with Theresa, her mother might think that the teachers are commanding her to take her daughter to the dentist. We don't have that kind of authority.

I postpone acting, not knowing what to do.

Miss Johnson asks what the sign for "health" is.

"I don't know what it is in American Sign Language, but in my home country it is signed like this. It means that when one is healthy, one also is strong. In my country everybody is strong."

We deal out papers and pencils so the children can draw what we have talked about. As the pictures are finished we will put them on the wall: drawings of toothbrushes, washing equipment, and beds. In every bed there are two people sleeping, a man and a woman! I wonder if the children are drawing what they see, or if they have a desire to find somebody close to sleep with.

I am pinning a drawing on the wall when Kenneth comes to me.

"Everybody strong in your country?"

"Yes." I swing my fist as if it's an attacking head—yes, yes.

"Deaf too?"

"Yes. Anyone could throw you out!" I can't help saying it because I have not forgotten what happened a couple of days ago. Kenneth looks puzzled. He watches karate films every Sunday. He admires strength, and, I hate to say it, violence as well.

Again, I don't know how everything gets started.

Kenneth is teasing Valerie, who is sitting beside him. With his foot he kicks the tabletop from underneath so the crayons bounce on the table and nobody can draw or write. And again Kenneth has the scissors. I am afraid that something will happen. Kenneth has lost his temper. I try to talk to him, but in vain. We could grab Kenneth by the arms and drag him outside, but it wouldn't help, because he would throw rocks inside or do something unpredictable. The only possibility would be for some sturdy man to come and carry Kenneth home.

But there's no big sturdy man at hand. The only possibility is to close the school for the day and keep it closed the next day. We can't guarantee the safety of other children when Kenneth gets his awful fits.

Miss Johnson writes on the board: "No school tomorrow."

We give paper to the children so they can copy the message and take the information home.

I throw chairs and tables in piles. I am angry. At myself, because I don't know what to do, or at Kenneth? I don't know. I feel like a martyr. Here I work without pay for these children. Don't they understand that going to school is their privilege, not an obligation?

Kenneth looks surprised. His rage is blown away for the most part.

"No school tomorrow?"

"No, and it's your fault!" I sign fast and angrily and talk at the same time.

"Your fault," Kenneth mimics; he apes my signing and lip movements, and it makes me even more angry.

"Yes, your fault. And I won't buy you any magazines or take you to the beach."

Andrew is collecting chairs. He throws them, throws the pencils into cans, looks angry—just like me.

He acts just like me. How childishly I've behaved. And my fury hasn't affected Kenneth at all. The other children are standing stiff and looking surprised. Can that woman really be angry?

But the only thing that affects Kenneth, the only thing he feels is a punishment, if he even understands the relationship between crime and punishment, is that sentence on the board: "No school tomorrow."

Kenneth has been in school more than anybody; he has been absent only when he was in the hospital. In a hard rainfall, when all the other children stay at home, Kenneth tramps to school. Somewhere deep inside him there's an insatiable urge to learn, and the knowledge that he *can* learn is sprouting.

"No school tomorrow," Kenneth repeats. "No magazines, no beaches. No school, no magazines, no beaches."

No anything. Somehow I get the feeling that he doesn't understand why. What happened half an hour ago has not happened at all, it was not Kenneth who took the scissors and got angry.

My heart is heavy the rest of the day. After school I lie on the beach under the palms and look at the sea, metallic-shiny in the sunset. Jukka also looks at the sea, thinking about his problems at work.

I ponder the reason for Kenneth's behavior, and a question keeps rolling around in my head: What could I have done? It hurts to realize I couldn't handle Kenneth.

I can imagine: A small house, a lot of people inside. On the floor, Kenneth playing. He sees and experiences a lot because he has a sharp brain. But around him it's like a wall, a cage—it's invisible, which is why it's so impenetrable. Kenneth has no means to express what is happening in his head. He has no words, no way to make those people understand him, or he, them.

But gradually Kenneth finds out what helps, at least somewhat—that he can make the others interrupt their talking, their work, and their quarreling, and turn their attention toward him.

He yells until their heads are splitting. Maybe it was by accident that Kenneth got his vocal cords to function, and he quickly noticed that this gave him a kind of power that he could use. And soon something else is added: throwing things, using fists.

"A child doesn't communicate only because he is alive, but because it is distressing to be in situations where he can't communicate." I copied this sentence from one of Clyde's books.

Kenneth has experienced many kinds of pressures—being constantly tossed from one relative to another, being separated from his mother, meeting a lack of understanding in his environment. The cleverer the child, the more difficult it is. I too have been aggressive in situations where I've felt myself in a communication vacuum. I wanted to throw my glass on the floor and run away. I just haven't ever really done it.

I understand Kenneth completely, but at this moment I can't feel sympathy for him. Kenneth needs therapy badly. Gregory could also use help, because he already lives in his own world, having established no contact with his environment—or because he has some additional handicap. I've tried to explain this to Clyde and others, but I haven't received any response.

"What can we do? We don't have psychologists or therapists," Clyde says.

That's true. We only have a few notebooks and pencils and furniture made out of rough pieces of plank and empty cans received from the bottling plant.

Every day I wonder what these children will be doing later on, when they can't go to school any more. Do they have any kind of future? There's unemployment on the island. I wonder if even the clever Kenneth can get any work.

And suppose these children want to get together after school? Do they have any need for that? When deaf people started to get an education in Finland in the middle of the 19th century, they wanted to keep in contact even after school was over. They founded their own clubs. I doubt if this group of older children could yet found a club. I think it's Kenneth who could most likely do it, but he lacks the realization that the deaf could and should keep in touch. These children have a long way to go to develop that feeling.

[handwritten margin notes:]
no sense of community

what explan. does Raija find for Kenneth's behavior?

IN SEARCH OF
ALFONSO

We usually have our dinner on the balcony at seven o'clock after the sun has set. On the floor and on the table the mosquito smoke-coils are lit, because without them the mosquitoes and sandflies would be having dinner—with us as their main course. Once a month a man comes to check that there's no standing water in the garden where mosquitoes can dwell. Actually he is after the *Aedes Aegypt* species, which spreads yellow fever. However, the mosquitoes are a pain in the neck, especially during the rainy season. Marshes have been dried out in lowlands on the island. Malaria and yellow fever have been wiped out, so St. Lucia is now a healthy place to live.

I take the plates to the kitchen. Zenia will wash them in the morning. I collect something to eat in a paper bag—a couple of rolls, cheese, some eggs. I ride with Jukka to the fishing port, and there I search for Alfonso beside the boats. The boats have arrived, but there has been so much fish that it has been carried across the road to the fish market to be sold.

The fish market is full of a cacophony of sound echoing from the walls. Big fish are being cut and weighed on stone market counters. Scraps from the cleaning stink on the floor. A man is shoveling them into a pile, but still more scraps slide or are thrown from the shiny, slippery counters. There are so many sounds, smells, dirt, scraps, and people in the market that I feel a desire to go outside to breathe. But I won't go anywhere, because the fish market is a part of St. Lucia. The best sight on the island is not Pigeon Island with its fortress, or the ruins up at the top of Morne Fortune, but the life that seethes in the marketplace, on the main street, and in the old parts of the town, whose beautiful houses decorated with woodcarvings were saved from the flames during the Castries Fire of the 1940s.

A man who works for Jukka steps out of the crowd and greets us. His hands make wide circles toward the counters. It always happens that we no sooner enter the market and stop to wonder at the swarming around us than someone comes up to ask what kind of fish we're looking for and whether we need help.

But we've come to search for Alfonso. I have the food bag in my hand, and I look carefully at every wrapping-paper seller crouching on the floor, but none of them is the one I'm looking for.

Our guide pilots us to a seller who is cutting up a big kingfish. Jukka starts bargaining.

"Do you think five dollars is a lot for that piece?"

"Not in my opinion. It will be enough for two meals, and meat is also expensive."

The piece of fish is cleaned for us, salt and curry are sprinkled on it, and finally the whole piece is dropped, modern-style, into a plastic bag. All this is without extra charge just because Jukka has made a good impression.

While Jukka drives I look at both sides of the streets in case Alfonso might be there. It's drizzling, and I worriedly wonder whether the boy is warm, or if he is wet, cold, and hungry. Or sick. He hasn't been selling paper for a long time.

"We should look at Morne at that place where we left the boy," Jukka says.

I've been thinking the same thing, but it's better that the suggestion come from Jukka.

The following evening, once again, I collect rolls and eggs in a bag. We have an hour before sunset. We drive to Morne and leave the car by the red clay ditch under the bamboo trunks.

The soil on the slope is covered with dry leaves and tramped down hard. We slip, falling, and barely make it to the house, gleaming in starlight against the darkness beyond. Chickens are squawking in the yard, but the door is nailed shut. Grass is growing on the steps—it won't take long before the exuberance of the tropics will cover everything left unused for any length of time: abandoned cars and old sugar mills, forsaken roads, stairs that have not been stepped on.

Farther down the slope we can see another house. A man feeding some chickens looks at us curiously and suspiciously. What do white people want?

"Good afternoon. We are looking for a deaf boy. Do you know if there is a deaf boy living close by?"

The man shakes his head.

"We brought the boy to the end of the path one evening by car. He said he lived here."

"What do you want from the boy?"

"We brought him food."

The reluctant expression of the man eases up a bit.

Still lower down on the slope is a third house. Women are sitting on the porch. One of them is combing another's hair in a ritual you can see all over the island. The hair is divided into many parts and braided into dozens of tight tails or twisted into small knots.

"They're suspicious," Jukka says as we climb down the slope. "They don't know why we're searching for the boy, and they won't tell where he is, although they know."

A woman comes to us.

"I do know a deaf boy around here, but what do you want from him?"

"My wife teaches at the school for the deaf. She would like to start teaching the boy."

The explanation helps. We start on the path, down the hill, the woman and two small girls as our guides. When we reach the bottom of the valley, we step over the stream where women are washing clothes. They seem unconscious of the risk of bilhartsiosis. It is the most dangerous disease on the island—a contagious parasite that can be caught from flowing water.

In the thick jungle we can see a kitchen hut with smoke puffing through blackened walls. Between its rotten planks I can see a pan steaming over the fire. Many islanders still cook their meals in these huts, or over a coal pot made of clay. A gas or electric stove is a luxury.

The dwelling house is farther away. A boy is pushed forward, from the house.

"Here he is."

"No, that's not Alfonso."

But deaf he is for sure. Oh God, how many deaf children are not in school, some because of too great a distance, some because their parents or relatives don't know about sending them to school. Clyde is right when he says that our pupils are lucky to be able to go to school. We have talked about needing a boarding school.

"Do you know that there is a school for the deaf in town?" I ask the woman who is standing with a baby in her arms. She could be the boy's aunt or sister, but she's too young to be his mother.

"I haven't heard that there's a school for the deaf," the woman says. Jukka interprets.

"On Monday at one o'clock the boy could come to school. Do you know the place?"

The woman nods.

To the deaf boy I gesture: "Want to come to school? Come on Monday. I am there. In school other deaf children. Nice to be together."

The boy nods and smiles. I don't know how much he has understood, but there's a look in his eyes as if he had understood everything.

But we haven't found Alfonso.

I'm still holding the food bag tightly.

"They say that this boy's cousin is also deaf. He lives with his grandmother, but he comes and goes, he is not permanently anywhere," says the woman.

He could well be Alfonso.

The girls guide us back. A slope goes up to the road where there are houses on both sides. Another road goes down, and we reach a rock fence where the road turns toward the mountain.

The girls stop in front of a house, gray with age, almost at the bottom of the gorge. The house is exposed to all the rainwater streaming down from above.

The girls knock on the door, but there's nobody home.

It's completely dark. We have to stop searching. I give the food bag to the girls. The car is up on the mountain, where we have to climb to get back to it. Our hearts are pounding and our lungs bursting—but if women walk up the mountain every day with huge loads on their heads, we must also be able to climb the mountain. And as we climb we look down at the valley, the town, and the port, and we admire the lights that wind up and down the mountains surrounding the town. ✒

why pick out one child to help?

ALFONSO STARTS SCHOOL

NB - the pen named Pen

T he midday sun is burning hot. The bright weather of January and Febuary is over. The sun rises even higher in the sky, and in the evenings it sets into the sea far from the lighthouse. The sand on the beach is so hot in the afternoons that we can hardly step on it. Plants are starting to dry out, and the illumination of the whole island is more glaring because the sunlight doesn't sift through thick foliage any more.

I stand by the road, waiting for the bus, but the buses come whenever. Finally, here comes the car that always gives me a ride when it's passing by. The driver finds room for me on the back seat, although the car is already full of women.

I'm late; everybody is already in the classroom. The window shades have been opened, and the fan is turning, up on the ceiling.

The girls greet me happily as usual. They clap their hands, come to meet me, and make my name sign.

I take my bag to the back room and have a gulp of water from my water bottle. Nowadays I'm always thirsty whenever I move about. Sweat pours down my face after even a little exertion, and my hair is constantly wet.

From the closet I take the notebooks that have "News" written on them. Kenneth, Joseph, Victor, Gregory, Valerie, Filipa, Theresa. I wonder if they all are in school today? Of course, not Andrew, who has not been here for some time. He has a weak heart, and it's a long way to school. Most deaf children on the island have just too long a trip to allow them to come to school. It's only thirty kilometers to the volcanoes at the southern point of the island, taking a beeline, but it takes hours by car to get there. Up, down, up, down—that journey can't be taken every day.

Raija named him

Patrick has been moved into the school for mentally disturbed children. Cynthia has not been in school for a long time; I've never even seen her.

I look for some pencils, sharpen them, and go back to the classroom. It's not until then that I realize that something special is going on.

"We have a new boy," Clyde signs.

A boy is standing in the middle of the crowd of children. Slightly curly hair, head held proudly—it's Alfonso!

But where is his hidden look and serious expression? This boy laughs with shining teeth, and there's a happy twinkle in his eyes.

I'm surprised. I've searched for Alfonso through rainy streets, even over the mountains and valleys, and here the boy stands now. Did he understand somehow when I asked him to come to school?

"This is the boy I've been telling you about, the one who sells paper in the fish market. Alfonso. Or Alfonso is the name I have given him. Do you know his real name?"

"I don't know anything about the boy. I'll go with him today to see where he lives, and I'll ask his name at the same time."

"Who will be teaching him?" I ask, looking nonchalant.

"You take him in the slower group. See how much he knows."

Alfonso comes into the group with Valerie and Filipa in a corner that is separated from Clyde's group by a plywood wall. Gregory wanders around the classroom. I give him a writing task and Legos. Later Miss Johnson will teach him.

Valerie gets up and makes sure that the wall between us is securely fastened, so no outsider can enter our group.

I repeat colors because neither Valerie nor Filipa remembers them. Colors, forms, days, months are the basic facts we start with in our school.

It's easy to teach Alfonso. Happily smiling, he learns everything I teach him. And even Valerie doesn't sign "bad"; she too is open to learning, now. Filipa gets excited and explains to Alfonso the signs for different colors.

"Look, blue is like the sky, and red is like the lips."

In Finland, "blue" is signed by pointing at the eyes. But you hardly see blue eyes over here; instead, we use the sky, which is almost always dazzling blue.

I teach Alfonso the hand alphabet. The children are taught from the beginning to combine letters. Alfonso's fingers don't yet bend well to form the alphabet, but he's laughing happily again. Suddenly he takes the pencil. Looking very important, he makes a gesture with his hand that means, "Wait, I'll show you something." He writes with clear and beautiful letters on the paper: *HAT*.

Very true. "Hat," I say, surprised. "Good, very good!"

The boy looks happy. So he knows letters.

Filipa goes her own way again; it's hard to keep her attention, to get her to do the lesson I've planned.

After forty minutes the group starts to get tired. Alfonso is yawning, and Valerie rests her head on the table.

Resigned, I reach for a puzzle and coloring books. I try to repeat once more the names of colors and the signs for the pictures in the coloring book, but for that day the children's learning energy is all used up.

However, the day has been good, the best in a long while. Eagerly I plan what I'll teach the following week. How can I keep Alfonso interested in learning and get Valerie to give up her coloring books? I've tried to be as encouraging to Alfonso as possible, because I know that everything depends on the first school days to make the boy want to continue his studies. For thirteen years he has been free as a bird in the sky; will he now get interested in going to school regularly, every day? He is clearly very clever. Even with my little experience, even in a short time, I can see that.

Alfonso has easily understood the simple gestures connected with teaching, but now I must manage to explain that there's no school tomorrow because it is Saturday, but after two days we'll again come to school at 1 p.m. It will be hard, and I have to ask Clyde for help so that the boy doesn't misunderstand and come to school in vain during the weekend.

As he's leaving, Alfonso can't find his pocketknife. He left it on the table when the boys were in the hallway for gymnastics, and now it has disappeared. I stand stupefied while Alfonso rapidly and vigorously searches everybody's pockets. The pocketknife isn't found. I calculate how many pieces of paper he has had to sell to earn the price of the pocketknife. His first day at school has had the worst possible ending.

But Alfonso calmly climbs on the back seat of Clyde's bike, with Clyde's rucksack on his back.

attitude

During the weekend I copy math and grammar workbooks for Alfonso. I have only one of each; we make everything ourselves. Clyde is always scribbling teaching materials. There are cardboard notes on the walls that Clyde has printed. Everything has to be visual and clear.

The children have words and models of sentence structures in front of their eyes all the time. Everything in the class has a tag: CLOSET, CAN, PENCILS. There's a weather map on the wall, with hands like those of a clock to show what the weather is like today.

On Monday Alfonso appears in school again. Clyde tells us that the boy's real name is Roger. Roger! I think Alfonso suits him better. I am used to that name already. Clyde says that Alfonso lives on Payee Road on the spot where the road turns toward Morne. So it *was* where we were searching for him last. Clyde draws a map: the house is opposite the gray house at the bottom of the gorge, slightly diagonally up the hill.

"In my opinion, the boy looks tired. I have to talk to his grandmother so she'll give him some strengthening medicine."

I wonder if it's the heavy eyelids that give the boy his tired appearance. On the other hand, I notice that he can't be taught too long at a time. But after the school day is over, Alfonso helps Clyde lift a heavy shelf from the middle of the floor to the wall. At least he has strength in his arms.

I am excited about teaching my group, especially Alfonso, who practically devours all information, smiling and open. And Valerie, who has completely forgotten the word "bad." And Filipa, who all of a sudden is bursting out everything she's ever learned, if only I have the energy to pick it up, because it comes out whenever, regardless of my plans.

Filipa writes something and shows me. The script is like letters, but the "words" don't mean anything. I have a hard time explaining that to Filipa. And Filipa keeps writing numbers that are correct, but they don't mean anything to her.

I try to explain the word "and." "Valerie is here. Roger is here. Valerie and Roger are here."

I take Valerie to stand by the board, then Roger. Valerie and Roger. Likewise Theresa and Joseph. Kenneth and Victor.

"No, no," Valerie says hastily. "You can't say Kenneth and Victor! Kenneth and Victor are boys!"

Now that I know Alfonso's name, I can teach him to fingerspell and write his name. As for Valerie and Filipa, we've written their names every day, but there are not enough days; they never seem to be able to remember their names right. They won't agree to write the same name many times. The same goes for Alfonso. He copies his name once, then he pushes his thumb forward on his cheek. This means "tomorrow."

The first sign he's learned in school is "tomorrow"! When he doesn't want to write or fingerspell or color any more, he signs "tomorrow . . ."

I am so involved in teaching that I've forgotten to keep my eyes on my bag. During the lessons my purse and the five dollars in it disappear. Again a body search—all these troubles, just because I never learn anything.

The money isn't found on anybody. I don't care about the money, but I would like to get my purse back. It's my father-in-law's old carryall, and it has sentimental value.

As I start out the door, the boys noisily bring back my purse, and Clyde marches a struggling Gregory by the scruff of the neck. So it was Gregory! Gregory, who so often passes me in town munching cake, with crumbs on his cheek and chin and a bag in his hand with more cake in it.

Clyde tries to get Gregory to show where the money is, because the purse that the boys have found in the crayon can is empty.

But Gregory looks as if he understands nothing.

"You stay home. No school any more," Clyde says angrily.

Gregory doesn't come to school the next day, but the following day he loafs back to school and mimes writing with his hands. He would like to write again.

"Out!" Clyde says and points at the door, but I hurry to say, "Let him be; he doesn't realize he's done anything wrong!"

I feel bad to think about Gregory at home—nothing to do, loitering in the streets with nobody to talk to. It can't be the right punishment for him to stay at home.

"All right."

But the children are all agitated about the theft. They talk about it for days.

Whenever there's a glimpse of somebody's money, they're suspicious and watchful, and they keep a close watch over my bag for me.

With Filipa I look through a children's picture encyclopedia that we've borrowed from the library. There are pictures from foreign countries, and history that children of St. Lucia have never seen. But Filipa has. Eagerly she explains for every picture: "Many, many, many. Far, far, near home. There are many whales, giraffes, and polar bears, and they have six, seven babies."

Kenneth circles around nearby; he has something to tell me, but I don't quite understand what he's signing. So Kenneth takes a piece of paper, scribbles something on it and gives it to me. He has drawn a picture of an envelope on the paper and written the words "KENNETH LOVE MOTHER $ 90."

Now I understand. Kenneth's mother loves Kenneth and has sent him ninety dollars in an envelope.

"That's nice," I tell Kenneth. Joseph circles around us the whole time. The boys should be out sawing and hammering a playhouse for the small children, but Clyde has trouble keeping the boys at work.

Joseph explains that Kenneth has a lot of money in his sock. That's all they talk about now—that someone has taken money from somebody else. A consequence of my mistake.

I'm sure that Kenneth doesn't take money without permission, not from my purse, anyhow. There's my bag under my gaze, and nobody will touch it.

I've forgotten the whole matter, but suddenly Clyde drags Kenneth in from the hall. Kenneth is fighting fiercely, but Clyde has a firm grip, holding Kenneth under his arm.

"Take his shoes and socks off!" Clyde is puffing.

Oh, boy, so Clyde has taken Joseph's prattling seriously. But I have to do as he tells me, although I'm convinced that Clyde is wrong. Kenneth is cross and looks offended. He kicks as much as he can. With difficulty I get one shoe and sock off, then the other shoe. And still another sock. And there, in that sock, is a sheaf of money.

It's play money from a Monopoly game.

The ninety dollars that Kenneth has received in an envelope from his mother, from the mother who loves Kenneth.

Clyde shrugs his shoulders and goes away, a little embarrassed. Kenneth jumps on Joseph, enraged. Kenneth has been hurt, humiliated, and what's worse, there's no mother nor love nor money, not anything any more. It's all Joseph's fault. Kenneth gets the rock that keeps the door open and starts to throw it at Joseph. I go to Kenneth. In a situation like this, only kindness can help. This time I know instinctively how to act. I pat Kenneth calmingly on his shoulders, help him put his socks and shoes on, talk to him about the book in his pocket. Kenneth dries his tears with the back of his hand and throws the rock away. I sigh with relief. We clean up and leave for home.

The next day, however, Joseph doesn't dare come to school, because he's afraid of Kenneth's revenge.

After a couple of days Alfonso doesn't come to school any more, either. He was in my group for only eight school days. I don't feel that I failed, because I know that Alfonso is not fed up with learning and going to school. He must have other reasons for staying away.

Once in a while during the next few weeks, Clyde or some of the children tell me that they've seen Alfonso carrying water up the mountain or selling paper at the fish market. Always in the evenings when we drive into town I look to see if Alfonso is near the boats, on the shore with a pile of paper under his arm. But he is nowhere to be seen. 🌐

PEOPLE OF THE CARIBBEAN

feathers along the Granny helps them see what they've learned

In early May we get our first visitor from Finland: Jukka's mother comes to visit. It's already a bit hot, and Nature is not at its best because the weather is dry. The sandflies disturb Granny as they did us in the beginning. Now we're immune to their stings, although the biting that begins every day after sunset is still bothersome. Granny can't sleep at night because of the itching. She scratches her feet, which causes sores that get inflamed.

We try out all kinds of salves, but nothing works except the salve that Peter Paul has brought us. The islanders use partly bush medicine and partly the skills of doctors who have studied abroad. Zenia often has herbs with her, and when I ask which ailment they're for, she answers only that they're for the "insides."

We drive around the island, and to my joy Granny is fascinated with the beauty of Nature and of the people on the island, whom she calls the "People of the Caribbean."

We buy oysters at the fishing village of Gros Islet. The village is like a small town, divided by straight streets along which there are tumbledown houses with tin roofs, a few new and just-painted houses among them. The village is encircled by a canal, and on the other side of the canal are Reduit Beach and the Yacht Club.

We've stopped by the village often and have friends there, three women who make souvenirs and sell them to tourists on the hotel beaches. For us, they always have beautiful shells that got stuck in the fishermen's nets or rolled to the shore with the waves.

Jukka tells the women that his mother is a retired nurse.

"Oh." The women are interested. What will help a cough? There's flu in the village, and some of the women have had a cough for a long time that nothing seems to help.

"Onion milk helps. Warm up some milk with sliced onion in it," Granny explains in English, pronouncing clearly and trying to find the right words.

"I've forgotten so much," Granny explains to all the people she meets. No, Granny speaks English well, and everybody listens very politely.

Granny could not have recommended a better remedy than onion milk. The women are all excited and drape necklaces of shells around Granny's neck.

One afternoon Granny comes to the school for the deaf and watches while I teach. She brings candy to the children and talks to them. Because Granny is a fearless communicator, she is very skilled at inventing gestures and signs.

Granny stays five weeks on the island and leaves for Finland with her suitcases full of corals, stones, and shells.

In the middle of June the island celebrates the birthday of the head of state, Queen Elizabeth II. Government House sends invitations to celebrations in honor of the day.

The whole family goes to Victoria Park to an old ballfield where big celebrations are usually held.

The members of the St. Lucia cabinet and parliament and the government officials sit in a covered stand, the women wearing hats and white gloves. People are congratulating those to whom the Queen has given honorary titles or orders.

With tall king palms in the background, the flags of England and St. Lucia are waving lazily against the blue morning sky. White uniforms and sun helmets, fanfare, cannon fire, parades . . . I feel as if I've slipped back into another time, a long time ago.

The first European to find the island was probably Christopher Columbus, who saw it through his telescope on the way from Martinique to Dominique. Later, the English and the French came to the island and conquered the belligerent Caribs, who had violently taken the island from the peaceful Arawak Indians. The English and French alternately ruled the island; it changed owners fourteen times until in 1803 it decided to remain with England, under whose reign it is now autonomous.

French influence is still seen in the Catholic church fiestas, in French names for places, and in the spoken language of the island, Patois. The last names of the inhabitants, however, have mostly been changed into English names.

In the evening, from the balcony, I watch the lights come on at the Governor's house on the slope of the Morne Mountain. Again we go and celebrate the Queen's birthday. We drive up the serpentine road to the Governor's House and stand on the lawn with glasses in our hands. Lights come on on the balcony, and the Governor and his wife, Sir Allen Lewis and Lady Edna Lewis, come out with the English High Commissioner. I guess the orchestra is playing "God Save the Queen," because everybody is standing still, striking a pose.

Lady Lewis is the patron of the school for the deaf. The Governor remembers every time we meet that I work at the school and discusses deaf concerns with me.

Soon the colonial era will finally be over, because St. Lucia will separate completely from England. This may be the last Queen's Birthday celebrated here.

Here on the island I can help make history by being involved in the beginning of education for the deaf and experiencing how the former colony gradually becomes independent. ✒

KEKE LEAVES
FOR FINLAND

I wait in dread for the first of July, when Keke leaves for home. He has to take the three upper high school grades in Finland to be able to continue with his studies. Time in St. Lucia has not been wasted for the boys—they've learned a lot of things that can't be learned from books.

Keke has chosen a career as a doctor, and the biology vocabulary he's learned in English will be useful. He will also benefit from having done carpentry, mixed concrete, laid bricks, and repaired cars. Joppe, for his part, is learning French and Spanish, pipe-fitting and welding. Joppe isn't in a hurry to leave for Finland yet—he can stay with us until Christmas.

I don't see much of Keke. He's either at school or in his room upstairs playing the guitar, reading, or writing letters home to his friends. Or he's swimming, in church, sailing, or at the chess club. He listens to records with John Eugene and teaches John math to keep him from flunking.

But even with all his activities, Keke is still close to us. Once in a while he appears in the kitchen. He fries eggs, makes toast, cuts grapefruit, squeezes orange juice—he has always had a good appetite. Often he makes chow mein and pizza for the whole family. If I'm tired on a Sunday morning, Keke prepares breakfast.

Often in the evenings we sit on the balcony and discuss things. The subjects are wide-ranging, and our discussion may turn into a violent dispute, with me and Jukka holding one opinion, Keke and Joppe the opposite.

"Don't tell me I'm just thirteen years old and don't know anything yet, because I know things as well as you do!" Joppe says, and I can see that they've learned much more than Jukka and I knew at their age.

*beauties, riches
of islands
sent back home*

The departure day arrives; it can't be helped. I watch Keke pack two big shells that we bought at Gros Islet. The second one he will add to the collections at school. I help him put coral in a box—also for the school collection. Keke dived down and retrieved it himself from a coral reef. He packs books, clothes, presents.

For our relatives, I pack spices straight from the marketplace: small brown nutmegs, whole cinnamon, ginger, brown hunks of cocoa. The scale shows ten kilos overweight. The bags are opened and things come out.

After packing, we sit on the balcony and look at the flamboyant tree, whose flowers have started to spread along the branches like flames.

"Why does it have to be so beautiful here now that I have to leave?" Keke sighs.

Anderson is also sad about Keke's leaving.

Anderson would love to write letters, but he doesn't "remember" how words are written. Yes, it is hard to remember for instance, that "Hahwahyoo" is three words in written form.

Keke has taught Anderson to write. Anderson sits on the balcony in the afternoons, scribbling in his notebook with sweaty hands and his tongue sticking out of his mouth.

Anderson likes Keke. "You always make me laugh," he tells Keke.

I promise to teach Anderson to write from now on, but I can't promise that I can make him laugh.

Jukka is away on a business trip. A short time ago he visited Trinidad, Curaçao, and Venezuela. Keke went with him so he could see some other parts of the Caribbean. Now Jukka is in Florida. He has begun a marketing effort for the port of Castries. St. Lucia's location is favorable for a transit port. Big oceangoing ships would bring cargo from Japan, the United States, and Europe. They would unload in Castries, and the goods would be loaded onto smaller vessels to take them to the other islands.

"This cargo transport would be gravy—extra income," Jukka says.

In the 19th century, big steamboats stopped at Castries port on their way from Europe to the Panama Canal or South America. It was easy for them to fill up with coal in Castries, because even big ships could easily come into the port.

The women carried the coal in baskets on their heads. For every basket they emptied, they got a token, which they then exchanged for rum in the nearby rum store.

Joppe is in school, so I see Keke off alone at Vigie Airport. I watch as he disappears, tall, tan, with broad shoulders, into the small plane that will take him to the Hewanorra Airport. I try my best not to think of anything. I've been here often, seeing Jukka off, and I'm always excited when the small planes, looking so uncertain, take off swaying and disappear toward the sea.

The emptiness doesn't come until the next day. I've enjoyed myself on the island, but now how will I pass the time? How much am I actually needed at the school?

Suddenly I feel as if I live in a communication vacuum. I don't have any close friends here with whom I can chat. I've hoped the whole time that I could find a friend with whom I could sit in the cosy Cafe Rain in Columbus Square or by the swimming pool at the Halcyon Beach Hotel. I know that ladies have all kinds of activities here: bridge clubs, golfing, lunches. Nobody has asked me to join in.

Actually I don't know much about what's happening in the world. We don't have a TV—they have bad reception here on the island. I don't hear radio. The newspaper comes out only twice a week. How I miss the morning paper that I used to read with my morning coffee in Finland.

A strange idea lurks at the back of my mind: I am a prisoner here on the island, a prisoner of the heat, of the sea that surrounds us on every side, of my life that is standing still. It is odd because, for the most part, I enjoy my life, and something new and interesting is always happening.

I would like to visit home. Right now strawberries and blueberries are ripening. I wish I could bask in the heat of a sauna on the shore, and afterwards take a swim in the cool, refreshing water of a lake!

Sometimes at night I dream: I've come into a store where the shelves are full of milk, real milk, not made from milk powder, and on another shelf there is brown, round rye bread, whose lovely fragrance I can smell and whose strong rye flavor I can taste even in my dream.

I realize that Keke is now with his old familiar group of friends. Sooner or later Keke will leave us; we'd better get used to it. At least Joppe is still at home.

"Keke left," Joppe sighs. He doesn't say anything else, but that says everything. The boys quarreled when they were small, but when one was sick, the other was completely unhappy until that sure sign of the patient's recovery—the resumption of squabbling.

Jukka is still away, and worries pile up. We run out of gas. How on earth have we been able to use up both of the bottles? Joppe telephones Peter Paul, who calls the M. K. C. There's no gas right now, but the gas boat is coming. The list of those needing gas is long.

If supplies run out here on the island, they're sold out for good. One has to get by without matches, glow lamps, envelopes . . . It can't be helped. This small island state is largely dependent on imports.

Without gas, life becomes complicated, but I remember the coal pot, the clay-brown coal brazier that I bought from the market for $1.50. And there should be coal in the closet downstairs, if only I can be brave enough to go down there. The closet swarms so with cockroaches that I get cramps in my stomach.

When Zenia comes to work—nowadays she comes as late as nine-thirty, and I don't know when her starting time slipped back from eight to nine-thirty—she starts a fire in the coal pot. Finally I'll get coffee. Over the pot, drinking water boils and chicken legs fry. A great apparatus!

In the middle of everything there's a letter from my sister-in-law Leena. Leena's family can no longer take care of our dog Jeri. How sad! What do we do now? The problem seems insoluble. Jeri is a big, strong dog; he can't be shoved onto just anybody.

Why on earth has Jukka stuck us in this particular corner of the world? Again our family is spread far apart. We only had a few years together as a whole family after Jukka decided to make his home ashore.

At school Clyde is tired, and I also feel that I don't have energy to drag myself there every day. I wish summer vacation could start!

"Note for mother!" Theresa reminds me at school every day.

"OK." I take a piece of paper and write: "At school we have talked about tooth care. Theresa has asked me many times if I can tell her where the dentist is, so I'll send this because she asked me to.

"I know a good dentist, his phone number is 2651, and his office is in the white house on the Square. Theresa is a pretty girl. I hope you might be able to get the holes in her front teeth filled before she loses her teeth completely."

The next day Theresa brings me a letter. "Dear teacher. It is nice that you are so interested in Theresa's well-being. But I would like to know how much this filling would cost."

Theresa's mother writes good English. The parents of the children in school are perhaps the most educated among the families, because they are the ones who have understood that it was worthwhile to put their children in school.

I answer that it costs fifteen dollars to fill one hole. I know that's a lot of money. The reason so many of the islanders are toothless is not only money but also ignorance—they don't know that taking care of teeth prevents them from becoming rotten.

On the last day of school we drive to the beach with the whole group of children. I hold the small children on top of the water, helping them float. We drink Pepsi and eat cakes. By afternoon I am tanned, relaxed, and happy.

When Jukka comes home, I light into him because he didn't tell us when he'd be arriving. But he realizes that there's something else behind my feelings. I tell him about Jeri, but I'm unable to express the homesickness I've suffered since Keke left. 🐦

"LOST CHILD" ALFONSO

All along I've had a feeling that when vacation starts I'll find out where Alfonso is. Is he sick or healthy, hungry or full? Is he being taken care of, or does he need help?

Once again I take a brown paper bag and drop rolls, eggs, and cheese into it. Now at least I know where the boy lives. I look for the note in my purse on which Clyde drew a map to the house where he took the boy the first day.

The house is at the bottom of the steep slope. Jukka has to drive up, turn around, and then drive down to the front of the house. The door is opened by a young woman with rollers in her hair. No, she doesn't know anything about a deaf boy.

After a while the woman admits that she does know one deaf boy; he sometimes visits them. Grandmother lives lower down on the slope; ask there.

How complicated. Alfonso was supposed to live with his grandmother in that house, but now the grandmother lives in the gray house where we already searched for Alfonso.

There's an old woman washing clothes outside the gray house. As she rinses clothes in a tub of water, she looks at us suspiciously. Angrily she explains something to Jukka—I read on her lips that somebody is bad and proud and has knocked on the door and then gone away.

We leave, and on the way Jukka explains that Alfonso is not with the grandmother; he has perhaps gone to his mother in the village of Forrestierre—the Rainforest Village.

"Bad boy," the grandmother said. "He came yesterday at ten o'clock and knocked on the door when Grandmother was asleep. She didn't let the boy in, and perhaps he has gone to his mother."

"Bad boy! Not true. Alfonso is not a bad boy!"

"Now, now, don't get all excited for nothing!"

Jukka doesn't leave anything half-done. We leave for the mountains and Rainforest Village, although it's already getting dark. We look for the boy, of whom we know only that he is deaf and is named Roger.

We leave the streets of the town far behind us as the car climbs up and up the mountain road. Down in the valley far away I see red-clay valleys and banana fields, beyond them the sea and mountains, and beyond all this the sugar mound of Petit Piton. In the other direction are mountaintops, and beyond them is the sea. We are surely in the center of the world, in the midst of mountains, sea, clouds, and rainbows; around us are rain and sunshine, mixed.

We pass a few houses, and a man waves at us.

"Where are you going? Can I help you?" The man puts his head in the window.

"We're looking for a deaf boy whose mother lives in the village of Forrestierre."

The man thinks and shakes his head. No, he doesn't know that boy. But Forrestierre Village surely is in this direction. Let's go and look! The man pushes himself onto the front seat and comes with us to search for the boy.

We ask all the passersby, including a man with a black book under his arm, who is hiking all the way to town for evening mass.

"The minister lives there!" The man in our car gets excited all of a sudden. "Let's go and ask the minister."

"No, we won't disturb the minister now," Jukka says.

More and more of the people over here seem to be India-Indian with features like Alfonso's. Have they been shoved off into their own village up in the mountains, away from the valley where they are hated, even though people no longer remember why? Has hatred been passed down from one generation to another? The Indians came to the island originally after slavery ended, when workers were needed in the sugar fields. Because of them, salaries have remained low.

We go to the village saloon to ask. Many willing information sources hover around us showing their interest, but unfortunately the information is not too sharp in their minds.

We must drive further, and we leave the village behind. It's almost dark, and I am fearful of our journey back down.

Jukka is tough; he gives up only when there's nothing else that can be done. The possibilities end when we come to the last house of the village. From there, we can only turn back.

The last house in the village, however, happens to be the school. The headmaster of the school promises to make inquiries about the boy and let us know later. Jukka is satisfied.

"Tomorrow you can go to that house where we looked for him in the first place. The woman there said that Alfonso often visits them in the morning."

I really don't want to get moving in the morning. I want to sit on the balcony and look at the morning sky and the glowing flowers, drinking my coffee slowly and charging my batteries.

But the next morning I go with Jukka into town. Joppe also climbs out of bed early, even though it's summer vacation. Joppe always get excited about things, and for a while he thinks of nothing else. This time the target of his interest is solar energy. Joppe warms up water on the balcony in various cans and bottles, figuring out a system by which water for the shower can be warmed by solar energy. That invention would be useful, because our small water heater uses a lot of electricity, and electricity is expensive here.

In town I give Joppe money for shopping, although I know that after a few days we'll have a pile of useless test tubes and plastic pipes because Joppe's interest has turned to something new. But at least he'll learn about solar energy.

I go back to the house we visited the night before. In the back room a woman is ironing clothes, and there's a big pan cooking on the stove. The breeze moves the curtains; the cat sleeps on the floor in the sunshine.

The young woman we met the night before arrives with a child in her arms. She still has her curlers on. I explain that she should write out what she wants to say. I'm looking for a deaf boy, and I'm deaf myself.

"The boy hasn't been around today," the woman writes. Her handwriting is good and her language grammatical.

"Are you a relative of his?"

"Distant relation."

I explain that I taught the boy in the school for the deaf and he learned well, but he suddenly disappeared. The boy is smart, and I'd like to give him the unfinished notebooks, so that he could do some studying at home.

"Teacher" seems to be some kind of magic word. With the help of that word I see the last of her suspicion disappear.

"The boy is selling soft drinks at the cinema in the evenings."

That's the most important piece of information I've received so far.

"Who looks after the boy?"

"Nobody."

"Nobody?"

"He lives on money he gets by selling Pepsi at the cinema and paper at the fish market."

"Thank you. Here is my telephone number so you can call me if the boy comes here."

"I'll try to get the boy to stay here; I'll call you. Do you want my phone number?"

"Yes, please."

The matter is clear now. There's no point in waiting here for Alfonso any longer, because now I know where he can be found.

"The boy is said to be selling Pepsi in the evenings at the cinema," I tell Jukka at the dinner table.

In the evening, on the way home from a visit to friends in the village, Jukka swings the car onto the boulevard. It's already past nine; the crowd in front of the theatre has thinned out.

"There's Alfonso!"

The boy is leaning on the wall under the huge movie ads, between the sellers' stands. I get out of the car, hardly realizing what's around me: the smell of food, curious looks of women behind their counters, slowly dripping raindrops, the smell of stinking urine from the alley, figures near the dark shop windows. I only know that my search has ended. Alfonso is there.

The boy waves his hand merrily. He looks open and without worries.

"Come."

The boy walks with me to the car. He sits down beside Joppe in the back seat without asking any questions.

"The boy can stay in Keke's room," Jukka says. I'm thinking the same *why this attitude ?*

thing, but the suggestion had to come from Jukka. I can't suggest it; I can't take the responsibility for such a decision.

Alfonso sits on the back seat, his open expression closing down. When we reach home, he has hidden behind his curtained look and apathetically does what he's told.

Jukka has taken command. Joppe and I bring soap, towels, old clothes. Jukka takes the boy into the downstairs shower and makes sure that he washes himself properly.

Later Alfonso sits on the balcony wearing Jukka's too-large khaki pants tied with a rope around the waist, and Keke's old shirt with its sleeves hanging down too long. I would like to see him properly dressed. He has beautiful features when he smiles, but today he looks like a forest troll. His skin and his whole appearance look dark when he's sullen and closed up inside himself, but when he laughs, it's like the sun shining. I noticed at the very beginning that there were two sides to him, but I don't think it's the same situation we found with Kenneth. I don't believe that this boy could snatch scissors or knife or hammer; he is not restless in the same way.

I felt as if I were living in the middle of a novel. A homeless, hungry child who is being dressed, washed, fed . . . I go to the kitchen to warm up some food for Alfonso. The boy sits quietly on the balcony chair. He has been taken from the street, washed, and dressed, but what comes next? We don't know, either. We've just followed some instinct, some inner voice, that has told us to help this boy. Is it a need to get someone to take Keke's place while he is fa-fa-fa . . . or is it a wish to look after one of the smallest? Didn't I already have this wish when I met Kenneth at Columbus Square? Kenneth should be helped by someone more knowledgeable than I, who can give him the love and attention he needs. Without this love, Kenneth will grow in the wrong direction.

I stir the pan over the gas fire, and suddenly I remember a small boy who is standing among other children in a big room. There are stiff farmers sitting on the benches around the walls, farmers who are looking at the children, evaluating them—which of these children can be taken into a farmer's house, and what support will the community pay?

That small boy is five years old and lives in Finland. His mother is alive, but too poor to be able to keep the boy with her. I don't know the price the boy brought when he was auctioned off, and I don't know what the boy's childhood was like after that, because I never understood well enough to ask the right questions. I'd like to know now, but it's too late. But I remember my grandfather, the former pauper boy, his eyes filling with tears as he looked at me and my brother, his grandchildren. We had a much better chance in life than he did—he made certain of that.

All his life my grandfather worked so that no child ever needed to be sold in the community house, so that people would be safer than that five-year-old pauper boy was. He served in the Parliament for thirty years, and in his own lifestyle he followed a simple peasant tradition. A part of my identity has always been the fact that I am Valfrid Eskola's granddaughter. I guess that's one reason why I'm standing here preparing food for this homeless boy.

Then I remember another boy, my father. He's sitting with another boy in a sleigh, flying over a snowy landscape. It's three o'clock in the morning, and the sleigh has been loaded—in the dark and crackling frost—full of carcasses. They begin their journey to the marketplace in town. After four hours of riding they are stiffened from cold; they pile the carcasses on the butcher's counter. They turn the sleigh around and head for home.

The uncles always have money for liquor, but food is not as important. That small boy is hungry, like Keke, like Joppe. All growing boys are hungry.

"Didn't you get any food in school?" The door to the cupboard snaps shut in front of the hungry boy. And what would there have been anyway? The boy goes to the cow shed, and makes pancakes out of the grain for the pigs. If it's summer, he catches fish from the lake and fries them over a fire.

All this my father told me about his childhood when Joppe and Keke were being choosy about some dish I gave them for dinner.

And here I have with me again a hungry, lonely child. Doesn't the world ever get better?

A DAY WITH ALFONSO

"alfonso"-compared to dog

In the morning I snap awake, aware that I have one more mouth to feed. I must think what I am going to give Alfonso for breakfast, lunch, dinner. With our own crowd that's not necessary. But now it's just like when we have guests—I have to think what to serve. I realize that now I can't use my vacation as freely as I expected, because I must take the new family member into consideration. For a moment I feel the responsibility weighing me down, but then I decide that one gets used to everything. It's like when Jeri was brought to us. In the beginning it was a lot of work—we had to clean up big puddles and piles, and we were constantly washing the rugs. It was January, and Jeri is a Rottweiler—a big species. He couldn't be taken outside, because his abdomen was furless, and he needed food five times a day, with vitamins like those given to a small baby.

It's funny to compare a human being to a puppy, but Alfonso eventually adjusted to the family the way Jeri did, later on, when we agreed upon a method of communication. Then life could fall back into its familiar rut, and taking care of Alfonso wasn't such a strain. But it took a while.

This first morning, I go into the kitchen, half asleep, to prepare breakfast. Through the decorative tiles I see that Alfonso is already sitting on the balcony in Jukka's too-big pants and Keke's too-big shirt. What else could he have done after waking up, except come where food was given to him yesterday? Maybe it will be given again today. The boy is looking around, at the buzzing red bees on the ceiling, the darting of hummingbirds in the flowers of the flamboyant tree, like butterflies sucking honey mead. Bigger birds sway on the telephone line.

I light the gas and boil the water, make toast, prepare milk for the cornflakes, split the grapefruit, set the table. I invite Alfonso to come in from the balcony. He eats a lot. Jukka eats his own breakfast quickly and leaves for the office.

"Toast?" Four finger rise. Butter, marmalade, cheese. I stare, startled, as Alfonso scoops his cup half full of brown sugar. What does tea that sweet taste like?

Joppe comes to the table with his book and eats two slices of toast and drinks a cup of tea. Joppe's diet is a bit unbalanced, but I can't do anything about it, or he becomes even more stubborn. Joppe reads while he eats.

Laughing, I point this out to Alfonso. Joppe always has his nose in a book, even when he eats, and always when Father is not at home. Maybe Alfonso will want to learn to read when he sees how important it is to Joppe.

After breakfast we go out on the balcony. My battery-charging moment with a cup of coffee on the balcony is gone. I feel that I have to communicate with Alfonso constantly, just as we communicate with guests; I have to say what we'll do now and how to do it. I no longer spend much time with Joppe; he has his own friends, his own business to attend to. The time is past when the boys were constantly asking me to read, to play games, to play with them.

Alfonso and I sit quietly on the balcony. He looks upwards, somewhere past me. He curves his hand and points to the bird that sits on the telephone line. Somewhere far away, in the mountains, there are a lot of birds. Alfonso signs eagerly. One of them bit Alfonso on the finger, the finger got swollen and hurt very much. Alfonso asked for a ride, the driver took him to town, a woman gave him a shot. There is still a scar on the finger—there, you see?

I note how Alfonso signs the concept, *woman*: the right hand makes a curve on the chest. In the Finnish sign language this same sign also stands for woman. It's such a natural, spontaneously produced sign.

Alfonso shows me his other scars, too. He has been beaten. A woman has hit him on the head and back and face, and scars still remain. I don't quite understand everything. Alfonso tells me about a baby, a woman and blows, of how he went away and lives alone now. Alfonso has pride—maybe a bit too much, even. He went away when he was treated badly. What he doesn't want to bear, he doesn't have to. Instead, he goes away.

I look at the scars. I am sympathetic because the boy clearly is looking for sympathy. I want to show him that I will look after him; I put salve on his cuts, which still look raw.

for whom is she caring when she cares for a?

I look at him, proud and at the same time frightened. He sits there with his dark skin and curly hair, speaking Nature's language. All his gestures describe Nature and everyday life in the midst of Nature. He tells me in his lively way about birds, mongooses, snakes, mice. He knows how to express precisely every movement of the animals: he is a rabbit hopping through the jungle, a dog dashing out of a gate, a cuttlefish stretching its tentacles.

The boy tells me how he has been cold, how he has pulled the blanket more tightly around himself when it has rained, and the water was almost up to his sleeping place. The cockroaches and the mice have walked over him, and he has been afraid. I don't know what he's been so afraid of, fleeing, peering over his shoulder, but he has seen—and heard—something. I think that what he's so afraid of are the old beliefs that he has absorbed as if from the air. What is his world actually like? A mixture of reality and imagination, close to Nature.

In the evenings the boy came back to his cave, baked cassava bread on the fire, made tea. He shows how he ate bread; bite by bite it vanishes. The boy's lips push out when he shows how he sipped tea. The boy tells me everything there is to tell about his life; soon there won't be anything more to add, because the boy's life and experiences have been so limited.

I don't know yet which old woman it was who fell into the fire and lay stiff. Alfonso shows me the woman's unmoving face, eyes closed peacefully, hands crossed on her chest. Alfonso has cried for this woman because she was good, not like the woman who hit him. But then the woman who was good went away from Alfonso, and he is all alone now.

I feel love for this forsaken boy. I want to look after him. Maybe I can understand him because I have more knowledge about deafness than the people with whom he has lived.

I look for Keke's old swimming suit and towel. Now we'll go to the beach; it's a lovely, sunny, dry day. These days are like refreshing oases in the rainy weather.

I sit on the warm sand. Alfonso goes down to the turquoise water, his long pants over his swimming suit! He has never had a special swimming outfit. He makes the sign of the cross before he dives into the waves. So the church he's been telling me about is a Roman Catholic one.

Alfonso disappears for a while, and when he returns, brings me a crab. The crab stretches its pinchers out, and its eyes are moving up and down at the ends of their stalks. Alfonso is always bringing me something: shells with animals moving in and out of them, leaves that smell of citron oil when crushed, beautiful coral. I might be able to read the black print in books, but Alfonso knows how to read Nature's book, and he's teaching me to read it as well. I realize that I know almost close to nothing about Nature on St. Lucia. I've been studying books without seeing what is right before my eyes.

But I can see that Alfonso would like to learn from my books. He takes a stick and starts drawing letters in the sand.

Right, this is A, and that's P. I demonstrate the letters in the finger alphabet. Alfonso draws the letter and I fingerspell. But sometimes I have to tell him that that is not a letter, or that the letter is upside down. I try to do this gently.

I draw the letters of the alphabet that are still missing. A man is staring curiously at us from some distance away. Let him look. I am the teacher, and this boy is my pupil. Let the man see that you can talk with a deaf child, that there are such things as sign language and a finger alphabet.

Suddenly Alfonso levels an area on the sand, draws a set of squares and in one of the squares puts a cross. I see! So now we play tick-tack-toe. Alfonso smiles proudly; he wants to show me what he knows, what he can do.

We play until Alfonso gets tired. We go home for lunch.

I show him that the bathing suit has to be washed, the salt has to be rinsed out. Then he himself has to go and take a shower.

"Tomorrow."

"No, right now!"

I have to start fighting against that word "tomorrow," and I sign "now" as effectively as I've seen Clyde do it.

Even Alfonso's bed is still unmade. I show him how the bedclothes have to be shaken out in the mornings, and the bed has to be made tidy.

In the afternoon Alfonso signs that he'll go to town. He says that he will come back when the sun is low, but it's not yet dark. I sit on the balcony and cut Keke's jeans down to fit Alfonso. The back seam has to be opened, the waistline made smaller, the legs shortened. Before this, even for very small sewing tasks, I've used outside help. Joppe's and Keke's pants are always altered in the store. So I find that a person can do what she must—when she wants to.

cultural misunderstandings?

In the evening I fix dinner and wonder if Alfonso will get back. He still acts as if he's just visiting us; he takes everything for granted, without thanks for anything that is given. And he knows how to demand with perfect ease. At the table he mimes drinking with one hand and says with the other hand, "You, woman, bring me some water!" He's like a king who is used to being served. This attitude surprises and annoys me, although in a way it's good that the boy has pride and self-confidence.

Maybe Alfonso automatically accepts what is given because in this society one takes care of others. There have always been people who have given to him, given more or less, beautifully or less beautifully, hitting or patting him, lovingly or roughly. And in this society the woman serves the man. I can't scold Alfonso if he thinks that I serve him and the whole male sex. But I come from a society where people are equal. Alfonso had better get used to getting his own water, and he'd better learn to ask for things nicely and to thank people in response.

The dinner is already prepared. The sun is only an orange line on the horizon, and soon after, when we sit down at the dinner table, it's completely dark. When I look outside I see Alfonso coming down the hill with a paper bag under his arm. Perspiring and hot, he drags clothes out of the bag: torn pants that someone has mended with patches. Alfonso shoves the pants and patches toward me, and once again I am annoyed. Without asking, this boy presents his torn pants for me to patch!

At that moment I don't realize what this all means: Alfonso has decided to stay. He has gone and fetched all his earthly belongings—which fit into one wrinkled paper bag. I patch his pants from now on. I am now The Woman Who Looks After Him.

Again I feel the weight of responsibility. I'm a little bit afraid of the fact that Alfonso has moved in to live with us—it's the fear of change. But basically I want to try and see if I can develop this boy who comes straight from the mountains and who has lived like a beast. He is almost like the jungle boy in the story, who has been isolated from civilization and from other people.

It is not the deafness itself that has isolated Alfonso. There must be other reasons why he hasn't had communication with others. Without communication he hasn't learned any language; without language he can't belong to any community. He became isolated and was left an outsider. Alfonso's situation is not a phenomenon only of developing countries, either. Even in Finland we have isolated deaf people without language who live helpless in the care of their relatives.

We have to find a common language to allow us to understand each other. I could at least teach Alfonso enough signs for him to make friends with other deaf pupils, so that he can feel a mutual connection with them.

common lang,
common cult.
common expectations?

they have none of these thing

JOPPE AND ALFONSO

I'm glad that Joppe now has company. Joppe has not yet adjusted to our life on St. Lucia, even after ten months. But poor Joppe must have had his greatest difficulties in the beginning. He had to attend a school that was completely different from his old school, with schoolmates completely different in their nature and behavior from his old classmates. They teach in English, of which he knew only a few words when he arrived on the island. Joppe now speaks good English, but in spite of that he hangs around at home, lounges in an armchair, reads and reads, and misses his homeland—especially now that Keke has left.

Among Alfonso's belongings there is a ball of fishing line, and by surprising coincidence, Joppe is in a fishing period. He is greatly interested in the fine casting rod that Jukka brought him from Miami. The rod helped after Keke's departure; it gave Joppe something to get his mind off his brother.

Joppe knows how to talk with a deaf boy. I watch, smiling, at how Joppe is gesturing. Through the opening in the decorative tile wall I have a good view from the kitchen through the dining room to the balcony. Joppe uses pen and paper when he can't find any other way to talk. Finally the boys leave for the garden, and because Joppe never cleans up after himself, the paper is left on the table. I am curious to see what Joppe has scribbled. Joppe understands that Alfonso doesn't know English, but only gesturing, concrete topics shown with the hands. Joppe never says anything stupid about deafness. Maybe the camps for hearing children of deaf parents have helped Joppe gain understanding. That's why I sent him there, so he would understand my problems as simple facts and would know my different world.

There are no English words on the paper, only picture language. A boy is

— 113 —

fishing. The hook sinks deep in the water. But there's a bobber on the line in the next picture. The bobber floats on the water to prevent the hook from sinking too deep.

Alfonso's fishing equipment is merely line and hook, which is customary here. But Alfonso goes and gets a fishing pole for Joppe from the bushes. The coconut-oil bottle loses its cap for a bobber. Joppe's fine casting rod is left in the corner.

"I couldn't take my fine rod, no way, when Alfonso only had a line and a bobber," Joppe explains later.

I sit on the balcony patching Alfonso's pants. This succeeds, though it never has before. What on earth have I done with Keke's and Joppe's pants when they've torn? It was my good luck that when the boys were small, at the age when they used up clothes pretty fast, the fabric was of high quality. Their pants didn't get torn before they became too small.

But even unexpected skills have their limits. I won't try sewing the zipper, and one of the pairs of pants is already falling apart everywhere; I won't patch those.

Across the lawn I see a dark head and a light one. The boys are fishing behind the stone wall on the pier.

When they come home, Alfonso has some small fish with beautiful yellow stripes. I wrap them in paper and put them in the refrigerator. They will be used as bait the next day, Joppe explains. Joppe is disappointed because he didn't catch any fish, but Alfonso didn't catch his fish with the pole either; he caught them by hand.

I give Alfonso his pants that I've patched and explain that I'm not going to sew the zipper. Alfonso asks for a needle and thread and sews the zipper himself! How much does Alfonso actually know? What is he able to do?

He seems to have mastered many practical tasks. He even explains that he doesn't wash his clothes in the river and doesn't drink the water from the river because somebody has defecated in the water and it's dirty; there are worms in it. I gesture that he is right, you can get a dangerous illness from the river water.

Now Alfonso doesn't need to carry water in a bucket up the hill from some faraway water pump. I notice that he's a clean boy. He enjoys bathing under the warm shower; he takes a shower every morning and evening. I give him soap and toothpaste, and I buy him deodorant. I tell him that the underarms have to be washed well and then sprayed with deodorant.

Alfonso washes his clothes skillfully. I watch how he washes his shirt—he carefully rubs the collar and turns the pockets inside out. He washes in the West Indies manner, just like Zenia, softly rubbing, once in a while flapping water over the foam with his other hand, in little patches one at a time until the cloth is clean.

But I have to watch that Alfonso doesn't soak his washing too long. Sometimes clothes lie in the water as long as three days. Alfonso says that this doesn't do them any harm, but I disagree.

Imagine from A's pt of view

"You wash now! Right now!"

Right now is an unfamiliar concept for Alfonso, as are *hurry* and *time.* Time is only the moving of the sun in its circle, moving slowly, no hurry anywhere. He doesn't have hours, half-hours, and minutes. There's no yesterday or tomorrow; there is only the vague "tomorrow" that means "sometime later."

After the first morning Alfonso has started to sleep late, till eleven o'clock. It's as if he were endlessly tired. He eats as if endlessly hungry. After breakfast he sits on the balcony stretching and yawning. He seems to be wandering in a fantasy world.

Alfonso's aquarium is on the balcony: glass jars and plastic bowls full of fish, small crabs, and other creatures from the sea. Alfonso dashes to the shore, looks around, and calls to us to come and look at a mollusk crawling in a jar or a fish jumping in the water. There are corals and stones, shells and green plants on the bottoms of the jars and buckets. Zenia is angry; she needs to wash clothes, and the wash basin is always full of fish, or Alfonso is at the wash area arranging his aquarium. But Alfonso doesn't know at all how to take the other person into consideration.

The whole life of the seashore is spread out in front of my eyes on the balcony in Alfonso's glass jars. Alfonso laughs happily when the fish eat the toast he has saved from the breakfast table. The fish are fighting, swimming around after each other, hiding behind the plants.

"That's a woman," Alfonso says. "Tomorrow, babies." I can see that the stomach of the female fish is fat.

Alfonso stretches and yawns and looks at his fish. He does whatever he's asked to—"tomorrow." But before he does anything, he disappears to fish on the shore and doesn't come back until sunset, when he can only go take a shower and eat his dinner.

Zenia is cross; the baby is arriving soon and that damn boy has taken her rest space, where she sits down in the afternoons before going home. And the boy could just as well sweep the stairs, because Zenia is tired, her stomach is big, and her back hurts. Zenia's objections make everything much more difficult. She is always complaining about Alfonso; I am always having to run after him and explain.

All adjustment problems prove to be mine to solve. Everybody leaves them up to me, even Jukka.

"Go and see what the boy is doing now. Tell that boy that he shouldn't do it like that, but like this."

And again I run down the kitchen stairs, explain and explain. I watch what Alfonso is doing, how he does it, what he leaves undone. I explain that he can't do it like that, but must do it like this. I try to find the gestures, I have to. But often my head is bursting when something can't be expressed in words. Everything has to be explained in gestures. Often afterwards I can see that the boy didn't understand. I am angry, and I'm more and more tense and nervous.

I don't immediately realize that I get tense and angry in vain. It's not until later that I understand. It's not only that we don't have a common language, common words. The essence of the problem is that we don't have common thoughts—our entire ways of thinking are different.

It is this different way of thinking that destroys Joppe and Alfonso's comradeship. That lasts for only a few days and after that the boys just tease each other. I suppose that teasing is sometimes brotherly squabble. But at other times it really seems as if the boys don't like each other. Joppe knows how to communicate with Alfonso; he understands that it has been impossible for Alfonso to learn English because he doesn't hear and he has been alone and isolated. But it's hard for Joppe to understand Alfonso's thoughts and reactions.

Alfonso thinks that he's always right, and he gets hurt easily. When the boys are playing checkers, Joppe usually plays according to the rules, but Alfonso follows his own rules, so there's a dispute. Alfonso lifts his head proudly and looks down his nose. It's hopeless for Joppe to try to explain anything to him, because he refuses to look at Joppe.

"When you were little, you had your own rules for games because you didn't have the background at that age to understand the correct rules of the game," I explain to Joppe. Alfonso is in some ways a little child. In other ways he has developed up to his age group.

I don't actually know how old Alfonso is. He himself puts all ten fingers up and beside that two more, but he must be older than twelve. Maybe fourteen.

What a strange combination of adolescent boy, proud and reckless, and small child who comes to tell me all his troubles: there's a lump in the throat, his stomach is upset, the mosquitoes are biting.

Alfonso's health improves in just a few weeks. His stomach gets used to regular mealtimes and varied, nourishing food. He shows that his stomach is satisfied and so are his muscles. In the evening he does his exercise, running on the beach to strengthen his muscles. Soon he can climb up the coconut palm and shake coconuts down!

MUM-MUM

My life revolves completely around Alfonso. He has to be taken care of from morning till evening; he takes all my energy. I can hardly remember that anything else exists.

One evening Jukka and I go to a party. Alfonso and Joppe stay at home together playing checkers while Jukka and I drive to the big brightly lit house at the top of the Morne. The large rooms are full of guests, and as we stand on the balcony we see the dazzlingly beautiful scenery spreading out toward the harbor and the town. It's as if I had come from such a dim world to this bright light that I have to blink my eyes. I have been so deeply involved with teaching Alfonso, so much in his world, that now I'm amazed to remember there is another world, too—polite, well-dressed, where I needn't constantly strain myself with difficult communication problems.

Of course I have communication problems here also; but now they seem to have shrunk almost out of existence, even though I don't speak the same language as these people and their way of thinking is very different from mine. Jukka doesn't always find a way into their casual conversation either.

My neighbor is a local inhabitant, and he tells me about all the dangers that threaten the island.

"Everything is possible"—volcanic eruptions, earthquakes, heavy seas, and hurricanes. Many times fire has destroyed the whole town. In the beginning of the century there was a disastrous eruption on the neighboring island, Martinique.

Our nice doctor, Dr. King, is sitting opposite us. Jukka tells me later what the doctor told his neighbor: "Look at that lady now, she understands everything that she is told, although she is completely deaf."

But I'm not the kind of person our doctor considers me and advertises me to everybody as being. I do have a hearing aid, and although it doesn't make speech understandable, it is a big help in lipreading. I can pick up from the lips the letters that my hearing aid doesn't make sense of. I don't understand much of the doctor's speech, only a word here and there. Sometimes unintentional movement of the hands expresses something.

I've often had long conversations with people without knowing exactly what they said, by grasping onto whatever words I could distinguish from the speech stream. Because some people want so much to speak the whole time, if once in a while I say something that shows that I'm listening, they're satisfied. If they happen to ask me something, I sometimes can't figure out what to say, but usually they hardly notice. Sometimes I have to say, "Sorry, I don't understand." I still don't carry pen and paper with me. I wonder if it's that I don't dare to trouble people.

Anyway, my reputation as a master lipreader has spread, and some people think that I'll soon be enlisted as a secret agent! What a danger I could be if my victims didn't know they had to cover their mouths, grow beards, or speak in the dark. Many people do that anyway, so I doubt I could be of much use as a secret agent.

I am no longer that poor, deaf lady whom people didn't know they could start a conversation with. The biggest reason for this new attitude is the fact that I do beneficial work on the island. I teach at the school for the deaf.

Sometimes I'm overwhelmed with doubt as to whether we're doing the right thing, pulling Alfonso into completely different circumstances from those he has lived in before. After all, he must return to his old life when we go back to our home country. We definitely can't take Alfonso back to Finland with us. We've given him the opportunity to go to school and develop, and when we leave, we'll try to assure his well-being.

But am I really helping him? Time spent with him hasn't been easy, and it would help if I were sure that I do justice to Alfonso by taking care of him.

We have to explain to our friends: The boy is my pupil, and he lives with us so he can go to school when the school year starts.

"You even give him food?" people ask, amazed. Food is expensive.

Of course we also furnish food. All that is included in taking care of someone. We've had quite a number of people, dogs, and cats in the house while we've lived on the island, and I don't think my food bill is any bigger than it would be if I didn't give anybody anything.

"You are good people," Peter Paul says. Good? I don't know. We just have to do this.

When we drive to town, Alfonso sits in the back seat in his new clothes with his head proudly erect. Out the window we see children in their ragged clothes. Boys are diving naked between the boats; women carry loads and have a crowd of children at their feet; an old woman is crouching on the ground selling paper.

I look at Alfonso. I wonder what he's thinking. Not long ago he was standing there selling paper in bare feet with his shirt split in the back. When the evening grew dark he returned to his little hut, hardly more than a hole in the mountain. He boiled water, ate some bread, slept, woke up cold and wet because it was raining and water had seeped into the hut.

And now? Alfonso has a dry, warm room, he sleeps between clean sheets, he gets breakfast, lunch, and dinner every day, he washes himself in the warm shower. He has good clothes, he smells of scented soap and of the hair cream that makes his hair shiny and slightly curly.

But Alfonso's proud expression doesn't say anything. I don't know what he thinks. Perhaps he doesn't think anything at all, but only lives a moment at a time.

On weekends we drive to the beach. Joppe and Alfonso carry the picnic bag. We eat ham rolls and drink Coca-Cola. The boys swim together. As I sunbathe I watch the dark head and the light head bobbing in the sea. The boys can dive through the rough waves for hours; later Joppe's nose is red and burned.

One Sunday while I'm swimming far out in the open water I see Alfonso walking toward the hotel shower. The beach is open to everyone; the shower is the hotel's, although we use it sometimes. Who could distinguish us from the tourists?

But Alfonso shows off. He has seen us using the shower, so he goes in, too. He stands under the shower for a long time, and water sprinkles on the hotel guests. I see the hotel guard walking toward Alfonso. Alfonso goes away, and I sigh with relief. But I should have known better! He goes to the next shower, with the guard after him. The guard says something to the boy, who doesn't answer.

He stands there with his head proudly erect, looking straight ahead. I know that he has escaped behind his curtained look, like a turtle into its shell. I freeze with fright as the guard fetches an iron rod.

I am far out in the sea and can't do anything; I will have to watch helplessly while the boy is being beaten. I am furious! This man will whip a helpless boy, one of his own people. The stupid boy! Why does he have to be so outrageously proud!

But Jukka has already swum to shore. He walks over to the guard, says something, taps Alfonso on the back and tells him to go away.

When I finally make it to shore, Alfonso is drying himself. Big tears are dropping from his big eyes onto his cheeks.

"Evil man," I say. "Remember, don't shower alone when we come here. You tell Joppe when you go to shower, not alone." I have a lump in my throat. What all has this proud boy had to experience in his life? I can see that this situation isn't new to him. He's been through it many times, and there has been no Jukka to prevent him from being whipped.

How stupid people can be! I feel as if *I* had been hit. I feel like a female tiger, ready to scratch the next creature who dares to touch my cub.

"When people talk to you, you show your ears: me deaf."

I have to make Alfonso realize that when he sees people's mouths move, when they look at him questioningly, he can't just stand there looking proud. The proud expression is irritating; it irritates me, too. I wonder how many times I, too, have misunderstood it, although I try to understand. Many people don't even try.

"You must say you're deaf. People don't hit if you aren't so arrogant-looking."

"What did you tell the guard?" I ask Jukka.

"I just told him the boy is deaf—let him go," Jukka explains. Then he adds with surprising violence, "Although it doesn't mean anything that the boy is deaf. When he doesn't *speak,* it makes people furious. And there's also the fact that Alfonso has Indian features. That's why he's stared at resentfully."

I contemplate what Jukka said about speaking. I hadn't thought about that. I do know that although it's hard for people to understand what it's like not to hear, it's even more difficult for them to grasp that speech is learned with the help of hearing, that speechlessness doesn't mean mental defectiveness, that signing is speaking. How often did I suffer as a child from having speech that wasn't quite normal. People feel uncomfortable when they hear the unusual speech of the deaf. My speech, learned early, is easily understood, but Alfonso has never been taught to speak.

We collect our things quietly, carry them to the car and drive home. The beautiful, sunny day is spoiled.

At home I ask Zenia if she knows anything about Alfonso—What people say about him, what his last name is.

Zenia doesn't know his last name, but . . .

"He is called "Mum-Mum," she says.

The boy who can't speak.

YOU'VE GOT A
NAME, TOO!

wants him to learn manners

Alfonso seems spoiled. Maybe it's his lack of training; probably during his upbringing, communication with him has been considered impossible.

I try to teach him better behavior. When he motions for me to bring food to the table or beats the table with his glass, I show him how ugly it is. I don't know of any other way than to repeat his gesture a bit exaggerated. Sometimes he laughs, sometimes he is hurt and big tears appear in his eyes.

I show him that he has to tell me nicely what he wants. I smile and rub my heart with my palm: "please."

"I want bread, please. Give me food, please."

Time after time I tap him on the shoulder when he sinks his teeth into his food straightaway or leaves the table without saying anything.

Say "thank you." I move my palm in front of my mouth and then downwards.

Alfonso doesn't learn to say "please." I let it be, because the children in school also learn to say "thank you," but not "please." Maybe it's too abstract to be understood.

But Alfonso learns to ask in a nicer way and not to demand when it's not necessary, because he can see that food comes in its time. When he comes to the balcony in the morning and waits, before too long he's being asked to have breakfast, and when it gets dark in the evening, he can come to the living room to sit. He can read magazines with Joppe, or look at the rainbow fish swimming in the bowl, and before too long he's being asked to come and eat dinner.

I pile a big portion of food on Alfonso's plate, because he eats a lot. Before going to bed he often comes to me and signs "coffee." The fists grind on each other like a coffee grinder. Alfonso learned this sign fast. At the breakfast table I point to the milk jar, to the bread, butter, cheese, making their signs. We must have signs in common so we can understand each other, and it's most natural to start with the names of concrete things and characteristics.

"Beautiful," I might sign to Alfonso when the morning is especially lovely and the sky bright blue. When Alfonso does something well, I sign "good," and if something is not good, I sign "bad."

At the breakfast table I ask Alfonso if he wants more bread.

"More?" The sign is made many times and when the lips move at the same time, it becomes "moo-moo-moo."

The next day Alfonso comes from the shore and signs "Moo-moo-moo."

I understand that he means bread.

"No, bread is not "moo-moo-moo." I show him the sign for bread.

I take a roll.

"I give you one roll, you eat it. Now I give you another roll, "moo-moo-moo roll."

Next time Alfonso has tea, he points to the roll. "Moo-moo-moo."

I get some coins and try to explain what "more" means, but in the evening Alfonso comes to ask for "moo-moo-moo." Now it means food in general.

I feel that I can't try to force learning on him. I have to teach him as we go along, signing simple things like the names of food at the table. I should teach only when Alfonso himself wants to learn.

Sometimes in the morning when Alfonso absently stretches out on the balcony to watch his fish or his lizards, I go and tell him that he should clean his room now, wash his clothes that are soaking, sweep the stairs.

"Yeah, yeah, tomorrow, later," Alfonso "says" with his gestures.

It is as if Alfonso is two boys. There is this sullen-looking, idle, absent "tomorrow" boy who suddenly disappears, and then this open, smiling, energetic "today" boy appears instead. In the "today" boy the urge toward activity bursts forth; Alfonso does his washing, cleans every bit of his room, colors many circles and triangles in his notebook—he does everything I ask and a lot more.

Because of that "more," I have to keep my eye on what he's doing all the time or I'll discover surprising results later on. Like the time he scrubbed the walls of his room with a brush until the paint rubbed off—and the room was just painted in the spring!

Or the time I came in and saw Alfonso's dark head between the lianas of the balcony. When I got there he rose from his chair and proudly showed his shirt—Keke's old one, which he had "repaired." Perhaps he's cut the sleeves and hem short with his knife; the hem sticks out, sadly uneven, over a stomach rounded from plenty of meals.

The boy has been hustling for years on his own without anybody's direction. He's made his own decisions in practical matters; that's why he's so sure about what he wants to do and what he can do. He doesn't think to ask permission.

But he lives at our house now; that's why he should take others into consideration and follow certain rules.

I understand that before he can learn and grow, Alfonso should have a feeling of belonging somewhere, a knowledge that he belongs to our family. And before he can feel he belongs here, he has to know who we are—Jukka, Joppe, and Raija—and above all who he himself is. But does Alfonso know who he is? He signs "fish," and "coffee," and "bird," but does he understand that the sign is the name of the object?

His name sign is a sign that he was given at school, the right hand in R-position touching first the left shoulder and then the left wrist. It's a little like my name sign, where the R touches only the shoulder. How impersonal these American name signs are—the first letter of the name just touches the forehead or cheek or shoulder; the place differentiates different people. In Finland, name signs are personal, they describe some individual feature of the person, sometimes even negative ones. For instance, Jarmo, who had a runny nose as a child, gets to carry for the rest of his life the name sign that describes a runny nose.

The name can be shown also in the hand alphabet, letter by letter. Yes, true, Alfonso's real name is Roger. He was in school such a short time in the spring that he doesn't remember his name sign any more. And although he has drawn *ROGER* many times in the sand or on paper, when I point to him and try to show him the Roger sign he says, "no, no," and looks repelled.

Afterwards I think: how do I know what "no" and the rejecting expression mean? What can they possibly include—associations, different understandings that I can't grasp? But just at this moment that repelled, arrogant expression makes me blow up. That boy doesn't believe that he has a name and that his name is Roger!

Angrily I collect the pencils and papers from the table and throw them in the closet. When I look at Alfonso, sitting with his neck stiff, tears in his eyes, I regret having lost my temper. But there's no use in explaining anything to Alfonso, because he refuses even to look in my direction.

I guide the stiff and reluctant Alfonso to the balcony, get him to sit on a chair, and leave him there staring defiantly into the dark. I sit down to write letters. Jukka is away. Joppe has gone to bed. I write one letter after another; secretly I look at Alfonso once in a while through the decorative tiles. The hours pass, and Alfonso continues to sit on the balcony, looking sullen.

It's almost midnight. I go to the balcony. Alfonso's eyes are tired; it's so easy to see everything in his eyes: defiance, anger, happiness, sadness, tiredness.

"You take a shower and go to bed?"

Alfonso nods and leaves. There's nothing left of his defiance. It's already another moment, he doesn't remember the earlier one, and he doesn't think much about the future either.

One complicated situation is over. I feel that there are always two choices: Alfonso leaves or Alfonso stays. As if nothing was sure yet—Alfonso is here with us, let's wait and see. But sometimes, when it's really difficult, I'd like to pack the boy off, send him back where he came from. And yet I know I won't do it. It would be losing, giving up. And it would also be failing, losing, if Alfonso left on his own.

Sometimes after dinner, after I've put the dishes away and wiped the table, Alfonso gets his notebook and workbook. I teach him letters in the hand alphabet. It's a long way to reading. The boy doesn't even have a language yet to read in.

I understand from the beginning how little he benefits from all this teaching. I get tired and nervous as I explain and explain and try to find ways to tell Alfonso about things in the little language he has, in his own concepts, in the frames of his own world. But I wait and hope . . . little by little the situation could change, Alfonso could learn some of my concepts and ways of thinking, there could be born some real communication between us. Our worlds are completely different, but they intersect each other somewhere. Alfonso is deaf, and I

— 126 —

am deaf, and we both need contact with other people, ones like us and others as well. I don't know which is greater: that which separates us or that which connects us.

Because Alfonso is happily ignorant of the limits of his knowledge, he has pride and self-confidence, and he thinks he knows a lot. He's proud of the letters he draws on the paper.

KJPE, he writes, and looks at me, waiting. He has a questioning look, he doesn't yet know words to ask with; he is asking with mime and gestures.

I shake my head. I'm sorry, but I can't say that KJPE is something, that it could be a name of an object or a characteristic, that it means doing something, that it could be a word in a language. How can I explain that letters are not an end in themselves, but have a function to describe sounds and form words that mean something. And that words together form sentences that mean even more than separate words.

"Wait!"

Alfonso lifts his hand to a vertical position. This means wait, don't say or do anything, don't go anywhere, just wait; I've got an idea, but I don't quite know yet exactly what it is.

Alfonso's eyes are turned toward the ceiling, and he's thinking of something, concentrating. I wait. Now! Now he remembers!

Proudly he writes the clear letters on the paper: *ADH*. He looks at me triumphantly. You can't say that *this* doesn't mean anything!

ADH . . . What could it be? Now it's my turn to concentrate. Of course I'd like ADH to mean something. That kind of great certainty means that Alfonso has seen it with his own eyes. But where has he seen it? I think of all the possible abbreviations, shop signs—but I can't grasp where he could have seen that combination of letters. Just to be sure, I look in the dictionary.

Finally I shake my head.

No, it doesn't mean anything. It's just A and D and H.

But Alfonso is still sure of himself. He jumps up and runs to the bookshelf. He brings one of Joppe's books, *The Conquistadors*. Alfonso often browses through it in the evenings.

"Here! What did I say'" Alfonso pushes the open book at me and shows me a picture on one of the pages.

Yes, there are the letters. In an old engraving of the town of Tenochtitlan, which the Spaniards conquered: A. Tezucacco, B. la Calzada principal, D. Istacpalapa, E. Mexico, H. Magistazino.

ADH, true, true; the letters are there, and Alfonso seems to have a good memory, but they . . . Oh, no, I can't do it. Okay, you're right. It's ADH.

It would be easier to start from the very beginning. Alfonso writes numbers and letters and gives them his own meanings. He is thinking of something while his pencil draws letters on the paper. The letters must have some special meaning to him. It would be so much easier to teach K and P and E and to give them a meaning of one's own and form words from them which then have the same meaning to all those people who speak the same language. Could I somehow match the meaning that Alfonso has invented for them, a meaning that I don't even know? Letters aren't good for anything, are they, I ask myself, if they don't mean the same thing to everybody?

Again Alfonso remembers something.

"*LBS*, he writes after devout pondering.

"Yes," I nod, accepting with my head and my fist.

I am happy that I can tell him "Yes" this time, that this does mean something. I get a bag of rice from the kitchen cupboard. Written on the side of the brown bag is "Rice, 2 lbs $1.20."

I try to explain what "lbs" means, but Alfonso doesn't have the concepts yet to understand quantity and how it's measured. I'll get my purse and show him how much $1.20 is.

But again Alfonso writes numbers. He looks serious, trying to remember, and then he writes a new number. Now he wants to show everything he knows and remembers, and there's a lot of it, in his opinion.

17568. Alfonso looks at me and opens up his hands, asking.

Yes, those are real numbers, I nod acceptingly. But I can't explain what they mean. For Alfonso they are just signs that he remembers. They have a specific form, and it's good that he remembers the shapes of the numbers, but they're only meaningless shapes. Alfonso doesn't know that behind these scribbles lies a concept of a quantity of something. Now he's waiting for me to show him a concrete thing that this number series means, but I can't do it.

Alfonso does know that there can be a lot of something, because sometimes he lifts all his fingers up, then down, then up, many times. It's his sign for the concept "a lot."

The American sign for "many" is almost the same. In it the fingers are slightly pressed into a fist between the motions.

I understand what kind of a miracle woman Annie Sullivan, Helen Keller's teacher, must have been. She was able to take care of the deaf-blind Helen's fits of aggression; she had the endurance to keep teaching her every moment. I don't know what to do with Kenneth's fits, and with Alfonso I can only be guided by my instinct, trusting the same power that got me to look for him and to take him under my care in the hopes of healing his deaf loneliness and equipping him for a better life.

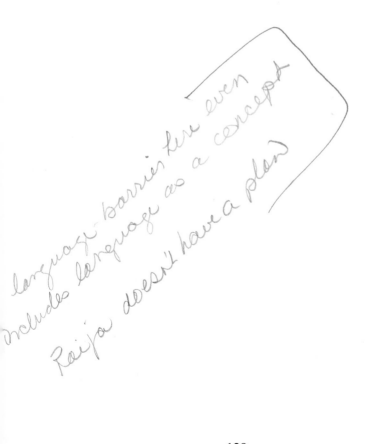

language barrier for even
includes language as a concept
Raija doesn't have a plan

HURRICANE WARNING

(handwritten marginalia: why this bk diff from others? place of deepness? whole family has adjustment probs)

Joppe spreads out sails to dry on the balcony rails, his nose all red after spending Sunday on the water. I pull together something for dinner. The sunny day at the Yacht Club has left me feeling fatigued.

Jukka is on the phone when I set the table. Usually I ask afterwards who was on the phone and what they talked about.

This time, he tells me right away—"I'm not sure, but I think there's a hurricane getting close to St. Lucia."

Oh boy! My knees go all weak.

It has been awfully windy for a long time. I've often watched how the palms sway in the grove opposite us. Their trunks are tough; they always rise up again, although their heavy tops bend down halfway to the ground. In the evenings as I go to bed I see the shiny leaves and shadows of the palms moving restlessly in front of the window.

Now it's hurricane time, and I have asked Jukka many times what we should do when the hurricane comes.

"Stay inside and open every door!"

Zenia tells me that when there was a hurricane, she was inside in her own room, lying on the floor with the door open.

I also remember a woman at a party we attended recently telling us about awaiting the hurricane. There was a warning broadcast, and everybody waited, afraid, at home. It was a horrible feeling, she said. They waited eight hours, but there was no hurricane. Finally everybody went back to normal, returning to the beach, going into town on business. The worst thing about high winds are the high waves they leave behind.

I have to do something! While Jukka is still on the phone I run out and collect the wet wash from the line. I lift down the flower baskets hanging on the balcony and put them on the floor. The flower pots, shaped like a man's head, stare up at us.

Joppe takes a pen, paper, and a watch and starts to observe Nature. A thunderstorm is approaching from the neighboring island. Rain has never before come from the sea; it always comes from the east, from the mountains. Behind the lighthouse the sky is bluish black. We follow all of Nature's unusual signs. I move plates and dishes in from the balcony before the rain cloud comes over us.

Finally Jukka hangs up. The hurricane won't arrive for six hours. Thanks to the satellites, the warning can usually be given that early, but not always.

Jukka can eat in any circumstances. Joppe and I try to eat a little, but we're too tense. I explain to Alfonso that there's a harsh wind arriving, and he observes Nature with Joppe, pointing eagerly at the black sky.

To the right of the lighthouse a red warning light is lit, with a white one under it. Jukka has called the lighthouse and the radio. He is on the hurricane committee and is responsible for certain safety activities.

"Now they're reading the warning on the radio," Jukka says.

The rain cloud from the sea is now over us. Cars are driving toward town in the pouring rain. Everybody is trying to get home to be safe from the hurricane.

Jukka is on the phone all evening. Joppe tramps through the lemon trees to the Barnards's house to tell them about the hurricane.

We sit on the balcony waiting. I take note of every gust of wind. It's dark; warning lights shine from the lighthouse. The red and white lights have been changed to the opposite order to show that the storm's power is greater than we thought, though not the worst possible. The curtains and the big leaves of the lianas are moving back and forth; the heavy tops of the coconut palms almost touch the ground and then swing back upright again. Warnings are being read on the radio over and over again.

It's nine o'clock. I'm tired. We go to bed, and sleep defeats tension. I wake up once in a while, but the wind isn't any stronger. In the morning the neighborhood looks the same as always. The houses are undamaged. The hurricane changed its direction just before it reached St. Lucia—it left us in peace.

A few days later the newspaper says there was a tornado in New York. The highrises swayed like palms, but didn't collapse. 🖤

EVERYTHING IS
POSSIBLE

One night I dream that I'm in a boat in the sea near the Pitons with Jukka and the boys. All of a sudden the volcano erupts and hurls a cloud of sparks up into the sky.

Afterwards I don't remember if I had this dream before or after the incidents that showed us we're living in a country where "everything is possible." First there was the hurricane threatening the island. Now on St. Lucia's southern neighbor island, St. Vincent, a volcano has become active. The eruption began as a small one, not dangerous, but the big explosion is expected any moment. Even in St. Lucia we're restless. There are demonstrations in the banana fields in the valley; the police use tear gas. The U.N. sends evacuation instructions. But nothing really dangerous happens.

Jukka leaves for Finland with the president of the Port Council, George Girard, to attend the Congress of the ICHA, the International Cargo Handling Association. George has a degree in economics from Canada and an important position as the head of the office of the Ministry of Finance in St. Lucia. I feel excited that George can see our country, the surroundings that we have come from. He will visit our house, see our garden where birch trees grow instead of palms, meet Leena's family and Jeri.

When Jukka is gone I forget the eruptions of natural forces, because there are enough eruptions already at home. Zenia is near her delivery time and is cranky. She doesn't like Alfonso and doesn't understand why we have taken the boy as our burden. Zenia is always motherly and friendly to Joppe.

Alfonso loiters on the balcony, sometimes feverishly active, sometimes smiling, sometimes cranky and hurt. He isn't aggressive—there's hardly any aggression in his nature. He just looks proud and defiant, big tears in his eyes, every muscle tensed for resistence, his gaze stubbornly turned away so I can't get any contact with him. If I touch his hand, I can feel how every muscle in it is tensed with defiance and repression.

Thus it is when Alfonso brings dark shells to me from the shore. He asks for an empty ice cream box for them, and says that the shells have to be put into the refrigerator. The animal is still in the shell; there's a round shield closing the hole. The shells are in the refrigerator for three days, and then it looks to me as if they've dried up. I take the box to Alfonso and tell him to throw them away. Alfonso is hurt deep in his heart. I imagine he meant for me to cook the shells, but I don't know how to prepare them. The delicious dish that I didn't know how to appreciate was wasted.

The toilets and pipes in the house are giving trouble. Many gallons of water have flowed into the garden. The pineapple plants survive, but the water bill will be huge.

Joppe happens to be interested in snorkeling, and I run between the house and the shore because I fear that he'll go alone to the reefs to dive. Joppe assures me that he always can find some snorkeling hotel guests for company, but I sit on the shore and watch in case an orange-colored snorkel can be seen anywhere. My fear is not unreasonable, because two German tourists have drowned while diving at the reefs of Smuggler's Cove. Yet I know that I'm overprotective.

From the time of Keke's departure, Joppe has had his classmate Stephen as his sailing companion. The boys take part in all the competitions at the Yacht Club, and because of his experience Joppe finishes first. Joppe dreams of attending the big sailing competition at St. Vincent in the fall.

Joppe also sails with the hotel guests. He has learned enough English to be able to converse with them easily. Sometimes I can see him swimming in the hotel swimming pool, chatting eagerly with an American or Canadian guest.

The days are beautiful and bright; the water is calm, a bit too warm. The flamboyant trees are still in bloom. I have time to enjoy this, even with all my worrying. Then there's a letter from Jukka. He's worried because of the St. Vincent volcano. I'm surprised; I thought that the volcano had died down. I've lived happily in complete ignorance of the danger that threatens us. I just haven't happened to be in town those days when *The Voice* has been sold. I don't hear the news on the radio, and Joppe hasn't been near the radio either. He's outside, and in the evenings the record player trembles at full force as he sits and reads and eats and reads and eats.

I ask Peter Paul what the situation is with the volcano. I learn that the volcano is like a bomb that's expected to explode. When it does erupt, its power equals that of an atomic bomb! The inhabitants have been evacuated from the danger area; they're living on boats in the sea.

One day Gayle Horley, with her small daughters, comes and fetches me to have a swim at the East Winds Inn. I met Gayle through Clyde, who plays American football on a team with Gayle's husband, Stewart. I ask Gayle what kind of effect the eruption could have.

"Earthquake or tidal wave."

We're sitting on the golden sand; the sea is a clear turquoise. In that kind of setting the news doesn't seem as bad as it would otherwise.

"If you feel the earth tremble, run straight out to an open place," Gayle tells me in a matter-of-fact way. She speaks clearly and draws words in the sand. I understand her speech better than that of anyone else here. If we had more time together, she could soon forget that I am her deaf friend. I would be simply a friend.

But Gayle is always in a hurry; she is very busy. She has a part-time job, she paints her house, and she takes care of her garden. Gayle came from Poland to St. Lucia with her mother during the war. She often talks about her father and Poland, and would like to see the country of her childhood. Maybe that's why we're so close, even though we don't see each other much—our roots run in the same direction.

"I'll give Joppe a call if something new comes up," Gayle promises.

I think to myself how I could escape. I should move the car to an open space.

In my home country I often ponder how deaf people can know about warnings that are transmitted only through hearing. What's the use of having beeping sounds at a construction site before dynamiting—they won't help if a deaf person happens to be in a dangerous place.

Let the volcanos erupt! I won't know anything! At night the storm starts to roar, and thunder cracks, but I sleep tight. I sleep even when there's a party somewhere in the neighborhood or an orchestra playing at the Halcyon Beach

Hotel, where people sitting close to the loudspeakers can become deaf.

Alfonso doesn't go to town very often; he seems to enjoy himself at home. But one afternoon he disappears, and by sunset he hasn't come back. I have dinner with Joppe; I put a chicken leg, bread, salad, and a thermos of tea on a tray for Alfonso. I am a bit puzzled, although I've had the feeling the whole time that Alfonso could leave us any day. Suppose he doesn't come back? Somewhere at the back of my mind, I think how much easier it would be without Alfonso. But I don't want him to leave. There's something in the boy that I like. At his best he is a pleasant, cheerful boy. At his worst he is something I can't even describe. There are good and bad days, as in school. As in life in general.

It will soon be ten o'clock, and Alfonso hasn't come home. We go to bed. At midnight Joppe comes to get me up; he wakens me, irritated, out of a sound sleep.

"Alfonso," he says and points to the door.

I haven't slept very deeply, because I've had a feeling that I'd have to wake up anyhow.

When I put my hearing aid on, I can hear for myself how vigorously the door is being pounded on.

Without hurrying, I open the door. Alfonso stands outside, ready once more to hit the door furiously with his fist. He looks awfully tired.

"Coffee, food!" he demands with his gestures.

"Oh, so it's coffee and food! Do you know, boy, what time it is now?" I go and fetch the clock. Alfonso can't tell time, but with this, it's a bit easier to explain time.

I show on the clock when the sun set, when we had dinner, when lights were turned out and we went to bed.

"You see it's dark all around already. You can't come home late; you have to come by sunset. And if you do come late, you still can't pound on the door with your fists."

I show him many times that you mustn't pound on the door. I think with fright that Alfonso will develop a habit of waking us up past midnight. It might be better to leave Alfonso without food, yet I go to the kitchen and get the tray that has been waiting for the boy since dinner. I understand his grandmother better now. Alfonso's arrogant way of beating at the door and boldly demanding food

what's to be done?

— 135 —

late at night is worse than coming home late in itself. The way he does everything is irritating.

But nobody has taught Alfonso. He has created his own values and behavior norms, affected only by what he has seen around him, what kind of feelings he has sensed, what kind of reactions he has experienced. The whole world is turning around his own proud self because nobody has ever taken him into consideration. There has been only himself, without name, age, or ties anywhere. No family, relatives nor mother country, no yesterday nor tomorrow. He can see pictures of birds and fish and fruit, but how can he think of things he can't see? He doesn't know what "love" and "giving" are, but he knows how to be angry and to take, demanding what is required for his own self-preservation. He knows how to demand, but not how to thank.

Alfonso can't conceive of complicated cause–effect relationships—*why* something is like this or like that. Maybe that's why he's so spontaneous. There's only his own viewpoint on everything. He can't imagine that somebody else thinks differently.

But to be honest, there have been times when I thought that other people were just like me and considered matters just as I did, and this belief made me very naive. My viewpoint is still, even now, affected by lack of communication. For years I tried to get by among hearing people when I was almost a deaf person. I had only lipreading to depend on, and it functioned very poorly, functioned only when I was able to concentrate on one person's lips at a time. Back then, without knowing it, I wasted a huge amount of energy in attempting to understand, when otherwise I could have enlarged my perspective.

How about Alfonso?

How can he broaden his perspective? And would he be happier? But the most basic social development demands that one take others into consideration and be able to imagine how they feel.

Constantly I wonder if I really am helping Alfonso. He has always gotten by. Does he get by any better by learning a mixed pile of facts, feelings, and needs that he might not have any use for in his life?

CRABMAN

It seems that I now have one problem after another to solve. If Jukka were at home, they might not be problems at all, but now they seem huge—for instance, the fact that Alfonso carries big crabs up from the shore. He spends many days on the shore catching crabs, and brings them home skillfully so that they won't pinch, just straighten their pinchers and extend their eyes on stalks. Without asking, Alfonso takes one of our trunks from under the shelter. He lines the trunk with hay and puts in a water dish that he has found among the junk on the shore. When Alfonso opens up the lid, I can see the crabs crawling at the bottom and on the sides of the trunk. The trunk smells strange, maybe of feces.

I know that it's not easy to catch crabs. I've seen crab-catchers with their bags move along the shore and dig holes in the sand, but I have never seen anybody find as many crabs as Alfonso does.

Alfonso is freely permitted to have his crab farm; the problem is only that the trunk will be ruined by the dampness, and it is expensive. Besides, I don't know how to cook crabs. They're caught for eating, aren't they? I ask Zenia if she knows how to cook crabs. Zenia shakes her head and says, "Uh-uh."

That's what she always says. Why on earth can she never say, "I don't know, but I'll find out"?

Alfonso understands that the crabs shouldn't be in the trunk, but where can he put them? He explains that he could build a cage for the crabs out of sticks.

"Let's give the crabs to Peter Paul. He has visited us every day asking if we need help. He brings us eggs and fresh bread in the mornings. We could give the crabs to him in gratitude."

I try to get Alfonso to understand what it means to be grateful, to give something for gratitude. I don't know how much he can understand.

The day before Jukka's return, I see to my joy that Alfonso lifts the bigger crabs from the trunk into a bag. When Peter Paul brings us bread, we give the bag to him. The smaller crabs Alfonso sets free to crawl across the yard; he says that they aren't worth cooking.

"Take them away!" I cry, horrified, but Alfonso laughs and gestures that the crabs surely will be led by instinct to crawl toward the sea, they won't stay here.

We wash the trunk well and put it out to dry. I sigh with relief. One thing is again in order.

But I'm mistaken. Nothing is in order yet. In the evening I notice that Alfonso is waiting for something, looking toward the driveway.

"Crabs? Eat?"

I explain again that we gave the crabs to Peter Paul in gratitude for his help; we presented him with them. I then realize that Alfonso believed Peter Paul had taken the crabs home only to be cooked, and he will bring us delicious food.

I keep explaining during the whole evening, but Alfonso continues to wait.

And when in the morning I go to wake him up, I notice that Alfonso has locked his door. I hadn't thought of that possibility.

"You are not allowed to lock the door. Imagine if something happens, how do I manage to wake you up, then? Remember, now, you are not to press this button to lock it, or I'll take the whole lock off," I add angrily.

The whole day Alfonso waits for the crabs, and I explain that there won't be any coming. When Peter Paul comes and brings the mail in the evening and doesn't have the crabs with him, Alfonso starts to understand.

He has big tears in his eyes again. Of course it's a bitter disappointment, when one waits for a delicious meal with watering mouth, and it doesn't come at all.

But I really don't know how to cook crabs! Or mussels, either! I've never even seen them before. I guess I'll learn little by little to fix these dishes of the island, but not everything at the same time!

From this crab story Peter Paul gets his name sign; he is from now on Man Who Took Crabs. Jukka is Man Who Carries Briefcase. Zenia is Woman Who Washes Clothes. Clyde is Man Who Drives Motorcycle. The name signs that we *onesick?*

make up are always based on doing, not on characteristics or on the first letter in a name.

Jukka returns from Finland, and brings my father with him for a vacation. Jukka brings bread, herring, rye flour, magazines, books, news. Now I can bake Karelian pastries for my guests. My mother has sent all kinds of gifts with Jukka, and Leena has been running around in stores buying the things I ordered.

Jukka tells me that Keke has started school and is doing fine. Jeri's care has been arranged. He is in the Katajisto Kennel, but Jukka will still ask about possibilities for getting Jeri to the island. Joppe could go to Finland right after Christmas and start school; arrangements have been made with the headmaster of the school and with Leena's family. And how has everything been over here? Well, there has been all sorts of trouble, but nothing serious. However, it's not easy to be here all alone looking after things. It's dreadful.

I'm tired of Zenia and her constant bad temper. Of course it's due to the baby and Alfonso, but still! I've told Zenia that I don't want her back after the baby is born. I want a maid who knows how to cook, not just roll her eyes when she should learn how to cook crabs or how to make different banana dishes to use up the boxes full of them in the vegetable closet.

But Jukka has come back. He takes a pile of magazines from his bag. Ten kilos overweight, but they're worth their price. I sit and read and enjoy Finnish dark rye bread. In Finland they don't appreciate how good rye bread is. The white bread over here is like cotton, it doesn't kill your hunger.

My father adjusts to our style of life. He does much the same as he does in Finland: sleeps and cooks. He doesn't know English, but he studies a few words like "beer," so he can go and have his afternoon beer at the small saloon nearby.

Often I see my father standing in the middle of the kitchen floor thinking what Finnish dish he could fix here: at least head cheese and pea soup. He stands by the stove, considers which spices to use and how much of each ingredient he needs. Keke looks just like my father when he bustles around the kitchen—they both take cooking very seriously.

In the evenings everybody sits and reads magazines, Alfonso along with the others. He looks at pictures and comes to ask me sometimes what the picture is about. I usually answer by flipping my hand backwards over my shoulder:

"Before, before," this has happened a long time ago. Or "fa-fa-fa"—this thing is very far away. It is hard to explain something that has happened a long time ago or far away, but still Alfonso stares at the pictures night after night. I wonder what he's thinking, what kind of images he has in his mind?

Joppe has become very active all of a sudden. I start wondering if it's still right to send him back home to school when he looks as if he has finally adjusted to being over here. But does he feel better because he knows that he'll soon be back home? The issue has been decided already. I usually waste too much energy pondering whether a decision is right or wrong. Jukka is the opposite—he never doubts long and he doesn't regret for one moment what he has decided.

Zenia leaves work; the baby is soon born. Joppe's friend John Eugene promises to ask his sister to come to help us. This maid arrives, and I realize that she is not John's sister, but a neighbor named Victoria.

Even Clyde comes back from vacation. He has roamed the Antilles with his rucksack on his back. He has visited Puerto Rico, the Virgin Islands, and Antigua. He has had only a little bit more money than was needed for the journeys between the islands, but people seemed to take care of him; wherever he went, he was offered food and a place to sleep.

If he doesn't have a place for the night, Clyde sleeps under a tree; he's not too demanding. He claims that he was in Death Valley once for three weeks to see it and to show others how to survive there. The temperature during the day in Death Valley is plus 50 degrees Celsius, far over 100 degrees Fahrenheit.

It's hot in St. Lucia now. Clyde walks over to our house because his bike is broken, and he hasn't the part needed to repair it, although he put in the order months ago. Here on the island deaf people are not allowed to drive a car. I wonder what would happen if I drove? I do have an international driver's license, but I have never driven a car here. Clyde is surprised when he sees Alfonso sitting on the balcony.

How did I ever take the boy in to stay with us? Do I also feed him? As I explain, Clyde reacts with astonishment. He seems indifferent to the boy's need, and to my affection for him. Sometimes I feel that although Clyde has a strong personality and is admirable in many ways, he sometimes is too deeply involved with himself.

We sit on the balcony and plan the following school year. At least in the beginning, I want to work a full day, because the children will be in school from nine to three, not just from one to three as before. It's not until now that they really start going to school.

There are also other changes at school. The local teacher, Cynthia Weekes, has been in Jamaica for a year to specialize in deaf education. Now she will become head of the school; the government will pay her salary. Another teacher is doing her specializing in Canada at the moment. The following year Nancy Niemeyer is to teach the 3- to 6-year-old children, Cynthia the older ones. Clyde and I will still teach our own children.

For the first time we have a teachers' meeting at which all permanent and volunteer teachers are present.

Now that the school is starting to be a real school, it would be nice for the children to have school uniforms. One afternoon is taken up with discussing suitable colors. Some people think that there should be a big label on the children's uniforms showing that they are deaf and that they go to the school for the deaf.

Why? I boil over. Why do they want to label the children?

But it would be an advertisement for the school. And if the children need help, people would know where to turn.

Of course that is the other side of the issue, but I still think people shouldn't immediately be labeled as "different." There are characteristics that label a person. Deafness can't be seen from outside. Only when it's noticed does a person get the label. Yes, you know that woman who's deaf, don't you?

In Finland when I sign on the bus or in the street, I am proud that I know the beautiful, difficult language. But in the past, deaf people were ashamed of sign language because it labeled them. They didn't dare to sign in the streets or in public places.

Well, if I've understood it right, the label will be put on the uniforms, but it will be small and not noticeable.

Yes, my reception of information at those meetings is a bit weak. I understand things if people speak and sign at the same time, but others don't always have the energy or the will to interpret for us. I sit and try to be interested and polite, as I think one should. Clyde, however, digs out a book from his sack as soon as people forget to sign, and starts reading. He can't stand any kind of vac-

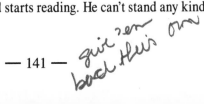

reaction?

your new

uum. He can't accept those moments when one should have the energy to smile and look interested even though one's own thoughts are all one has to be interested in.

I can't take a book out of my bag and start reading when I go somewhere with Jukka. I can't demonstrate the way Clyde does: As it seems you don't want to sign, I don't want to look at your mouths, which from my point of view are chewing on nonsense.

Often after a couple of hours I've had enough. I can tell Jukka—with a radiant smile, in Finnish, which nobody understands over here—"Miserable situation! I can't take it any more; let's go home."

And Jukka answers, just as smilingly, "We can't leave quite yet—I'm sorry. Go and take a walk and look around a bit."

Sometimes there are situations when you can't do anything at all—can't take pen and paper from the bag, can't find any good communicators around, can't find anything to look at. There really is no perfect solution to this problem.

life isn't perfect

SENIOR CLASS

I am excited and wait for Monday, the first day of school. But when Monday arrives, I'm tired and depressed, because on Sunday everything goes wrong. We go to the Yacht Club for lunch, and Alfonso can't go in torn pants. I've waited to see what the new school uniform will be like before I buy him new clothes. Keke's old jeans can do for school pants at first. I've explained this to Alfonso: These pants are for school. School starts tomorrow.

Sunday morning, I tell Alfonso, "Change clothes. We go eat. Wear these jeans, and that shirt."

"No," he says determinedly. "Tomorrow these pants to school. Not to shore."

"But we go eat now. People look at you. Must have clean pants."

No. Alfonso gazes again toward some distant place and has curtained his eyes. He looks as if he won't give in.

"When you live with us, you do as you are told. If not, you don't live here!" In the face of Alfonso's determination I am weak; I can't help blowing up.

"If you don't change your clothes, you can't come along!"

What does Alfonso understand from this?

One thing is clear to him: Tomorrow school starts, and that's when clean jeans are put on. But for me it's clear that Alfonso has to change clothes if he wants to go with us. I leave him to think it over.

I don't know how Alfonso has understood the matter, but when I go and see, _X_ Alfonso has collected his clothes in a bag. A paper bagful of property.

Is it now that it happens? And for this kind of reason? _clash of wills_

"Alfonso has collected all his clothes in a bag. He'd rather leave than change clothes," I say worriedly to Jukka.

"Let him go then," Jukka says. "We won't force him to stay."

But we decide that we can't give in yet. It might be that Alfonso has misunderstood me, thought that he has to leave if he doesn't change clothes.

Jukka goes downstairs. His forefinger speaks more effectively than any of my gestures. I wonder if I explain in a too complicated way, use expressions that are too abstract?

"Bag away. Those pants on."

Faced with Jukka's gestures—which no one can possibly misinterpret, they speak so clearly—even Alfonso can't say "No."

After a while Alfonso comes from his room with the jeans on. Soon he has forgotten the whole matter. But these kinds of incidents are never completely random, I'm gradually noticing. There are days when everything goes well, and days when all Alfonso's defiance, pride, and obstinacy come out. I have figured out that these bad days come when Alfonso has had it nice and comfortable, when he has been waited on, when he has received something, when he has been treated like a family member. Everything seems to go better when we are strict toward Alfonso all the time, don't let him take food from the fridge, and don't take him everywhere. He responds to our goodness by being crudely pompous and triumphant.

I've started to grasp this, but I can't understand it. I expected Alfonso to feel grateful for what we give him, to respond to goodness with goodness, and to love with love. Now it seems to be quite the opposite.

We drive to the Yacht Club. I don't know what people there think when Alfonso is with us.

I sit in the shade and watch the sailors push their boats out over the waves rolling in to shore and then jump in the boat. Soon the bay in front of Pigeon Island is full of brightly colored sails. I watch them all day. Father walks or stands on the hot sand. He wants to become "completely black," and surely he will, but how does his head stand that hot sun?

You can walk for miles on the shore. On the other side of the Yacht Club there are parties or picnics; a bit farther along there's the Holiday Inn. Boats are sailing along the canal to the Rodney Bay Yacht Port. Sailors from all over the world come here. They stop in Castries Port or Marigot Bay, or here in Rodney Bay, during their Caribbean sail.

We've met a couple of Finnish sailors who sold their properties back home, bought a sailboat and now live here, by the sea, in the warmth and sunshine. They find out that the port director is a Finnish sea captain, and they come to greet him at the Port Office.

For lunch we have turkey and salad on the beach. The women at the Yacht Club prepare the lunch. When it was my turn to help, my task was to cook a big kettleful of rice.

In the afternoon Joppe collects the sails and cleans up the boat, with help from all of us. The sun has already dropped a bit lower; it's the best moment of the day to be on the beach. My skin feels burned, even though I sat in the shade. The sun's rays reflect strongly from the sea.

When we come home, Jukka and Joppe start washing the car.

Alfonso says that he will go to the movies.

"No, Alfonso doesn't go to the movies now. We go to bed early; tomorrow is the first day of school. Alfonso comes here and helps Jukka with the car washing."

I show Alfonso how low the sun already is. Soon it will set. Then we eat and go to bed. In the morning we wake up early and go to school.

"I go to movies," Alfonso signs, standing on the balcony defiantly. He watches Joppe put the sponge in the foaming water and wash the dust off the car.

"No, you don't go. You stay at home. Now you go down and wash the car. Joppe washes the car, and Alfonso washes the car. No movies. The sun sets soon, and it will be dark."

"Give me key and pants. I go to movies." Alfonso smiles, looking at me mockingly, as always when he thinks I am talking nonsense and he himself knows absolutely and far better than I what is right.

I light the mosquito coils, because after sunset the mosquitoes start their stinging. I set the teacups on the balcony table and water the flowers.

When I look up the road, I see Alfonso striding along with determined steps. He's wearing his old pants and an old shirt—and usually the gentleman doesn't leave for town except in his best! Once in a while he glances back.

"I go to the movies when I want to. Just try and stop me!" his expression says. He has left without permission, against Jukka's orders, against his "father's" will. But what does Alfonso understand about family and father? He has never had a father telling him what to do or what not to do. I've tried to explain to Alfonso about "family," "father," and "mother." I've shown him our family picture. I've drawn a house, man, woman, children. Look now. This is father. He works and gets money, and then mother buys food. These are children. All live in a house and help each other. The children do as the father tells them. I don't realize that I'm presenting Alfonso with a model of a family that can't be seen in this society—few families here have a father. The mother is the power figure, who both obtains the food and looks after the family.

Jukka awakens me from a sound sleep.

"Alfonso!" Jukka says angrily.

Alfonso is fiercely pounding on the door. We go and open it.

Jukka's language is short and pithy: the forefinger points at the clock and at the dark night. It points at the door and moves threateningly in front of Alfonso's nose: that door won't be pounded on again. The hand grasps Alfonso's tousled hair. We are not in favor of corporal punishment, but in this case it's the best possible message, so that Alfonso will remember better than from any signs. Finally the forefinger points Alfonso to his room and his bed. And there is no mention of a meal.

"You coddle that boy too much."

Yes, I guess I coddle him. But if you're a caring type and a mother hen, it can't be helped. And yet Jukka is right; it isn't good to wait on the boy too much.

Alfonso goes to his room a humble boy.

I can't sleep very well that night. In the morning I'm tired and nervous—I spent the previous day and night fighting with Alfonso! Besides that, I am worried about how everything will go in school, how the proud Alfonso might react if Kenneth teases him about his ignorance. Kenneth wouldn't think, wouldn't realize that Alfonso has been in school only eight days in his life. How can Alfonso sit for six hours a day in school when most of the topics are strange and the other children are much further ahead?

On top of everything else there's my worry about whether I can ever get Alfonso to adjust to our way of life. I haven't been able to find a common language with him no matter how hard I've tried. Even Jukka has found better

— 146 —

means to make Alfonso understand. Everything seems so hopeless.

"Ask Clyde to explain everything to that boy once and for all," Jukka says when he opens the car door for us in front of the school.

It's still early. I stand in front of the schoolhouse, downhearted. Alfonso stands a little farther away. We're waiting for Clyde and the children. I'm glad Clyde comes a little early, so I can tell him my troubles.

Clyde informs Alfonso that Raija is "mother" now, who takes care of him. Isn't Alfonso happy that he gets everything from Raija and Raija's husband? And where would Alfonso go if he was not at Raija's?

Alfonso smiles scornfully.

He would go "home" by car (a square one, he indicates). No he doesn't want to thank Raija, and there's nothing to be thankful for.

I feel beaten. Clyde spreads his hands, shrugs his shoulders, shakes his head . . . and goes away. I swallow my sobs. The children start to arrive. Like a forest fire the information spreads that Alfonso lives with us, has for weeks.

All the children are crowded around me making the signs "Roger," and "home," and "Raija." Does Roger really live with Raija? Many of them would also like to live at my house. "Yes, he lives with me," I answer submissively.

I watch Alfonso the whole day, out of the corner of my eye, and see how he smiles his best smile. I imagine he's enjoying himself. During the lunch break I push a few sandwiches to him. They have chopped egg in them. Alfonso has a new drinking bottle that I've filled with juice. But what is all this worth? All my willingness to help is taken for granted.

In the afternoon after school I take my bag and go to the bus stop without saying anything to Alfonso. He can go "home" now, I don't have the energy to try again.

But Alfonso follows a little distance behind me, as small children run from the yard and sign again asking "Roger?" Does Roger really live at my house? I stop at the bakery to buy bread. As we approach the bus stop, I sign to Alfonso that he should ride up on top. I go into the shelter beside the driver. The other children must walk all the way home. Joseph's home is another couple of miles farther than ours.

People look at us when we get off the bus. What is a black boy doing with a white woman? Carrying her bags or what?

We walk up the hill and down the other hill home. I have my work along with me even at home; I don't get rid of it at three o'clock in the afternoon, it follows me like a shadow. And at home I have to be lively in the company of Jukka, Joppe, and my father. A dinner has to be served, and the evening tea, and in the morning I have to fill lunchboxes for three and prepare breakfast.

The kitchen door is open, and I see Victoria working. All of a sudden I notice how hot the afternoon is. The kitchen is a mess, and none of the floors have been swept in the whole house. The fridge is puffing in the hot sunshine that streams through the kitchen doorway.

"Dinner?"

Victoria opens the oven door. There are five fried herring-sized fish and a few breadfruit balls, to serve five people.

Doubt starts creeping into my mind about what will come of this. Have I taken on too much and not safeguarded my strength? Is depression and tiredness the only result of my work?

At school things are improving, thanks to growing support from the government and greater aid from different societies. There are three classes in the school now: something new is the "reception class" for very young children. Some still have a milk bottle with them, and they take a nap in the afternoon. The "infant class" is for younger children who have been at school for a year or two.

The reception class and the infant class are in the building where all the children were during the previous year. There are two big blackboards in the classroom. The little board from which the chalk ledge kept falling on the floor has finally been thrown away, I guess. We've received some old desks that have been painted light green.

Our pupils are now in the "senior" class, in a completely different building which is owned by the Red Cross. There is also a huge blackboard in our classroom, and we now have a big table that's the right height, and enough chairs for everyone.

I look at Kenneth, Joseph, Victor, Theresa, Filipa, and Valerie, and I wonder. What has happened to them during the vacation? They've changed, or does it only feel like it because the setting is different? No, they really have changed.

Filipa, who is fastest in growing up to be a woman, flutters her eyelashes more than before. Her mouth is puckered and held slightly open like a photo model's. Filipa throws long glances to Victor, who is sitting on the other side of the table.

Our pupils are starting to be young men and women. We can't actually call them children any more. But they're our children as long as they're in school; we can't help thinking of them that way.

From somewhere there has appeared a faint idea of being en rapport. Our students seem to have ripened enough to acquire the sense of community that we've been trying to teach them. Is this really the same disorganized, uncooperative, teasing, sometimes even aggressive group? Where have this rapport and all these beautiful manners come from during the short vacation? It's hard to explain. Has all the knowledge sort of hatched out from somewhere? What was taught hasn't flowed away like water off a duck's back—part of it sank into the subconscious, and it's popping out now. These children have reached a level of maturity at which they can act in the ways we've been teaching them.

How often have they been told "Thank you, say thank you"—by example, by reminding, by tapping on the shoulder: "Look now, like this, *thank you.*"

Now suddenly it seems as if they'd invented the whole thing themselves. The hand flies forward from the lips: "Thank you!" And if it's forgotten once in a while, the oversight is corrected right away. Sometimes we need to remind them that they also should thank each other, not just Clyde and me.

If somebody signs impatiently to someone else: "Pass that glue over here," I remind them: "Why do you ask for it like that? You can smile and sign 'please,' can't you?" They seem to understand, and they remember.

Victor's *thank you* is as smooth as Victor's whole behavior, if a bit exaggerated. He is manifesting himself as a dancer and an actor. In thanking, his hand flies out in a big circle. Soon the others take up Victor's exaggerated way of thanking, so that now "thank you" really can be seen!

One morning when Alfonso has finished his breakfast, he takes the dishes into the kitchen and swings his hand in a big circle for thanks. I look at him surprised and happy. Alfonso understands that I am happy; when I go through the kitchen door he stares at me. Between us a contact is born all of a sudden, for a *adaption?.*

neatly?,

short moment: Alfonso at his best. He is beautiful and smiling, he has had a good breakfast, taken a shower, is leaving for school—he is our son, he is satisfied; I am satisfied with him, and we both know it.

It appears that my teaching has borne fruit. School helps a lot with Alfonso's behavior. When I teach him something at home, it is often too new for him, like thanking. For him the concept of thanking never before existed. Now, at school, he can see that it isn't some casual matter that only belongs to our house. Everybody in school thanks. He does the same without noticing it.

I start to grasp that there's no point in demanding anything from a child too early. If he isn't mature enough to learn something, there's no point in expecting him to learn. But in Alfonso's case it's impossible to know when the time is ripe. He isn't an average child who fits the definition of when a child learns this or that. No, he is a wonderful mixture of a child at different developmental levels; the rules made for our culture don't fit him.

hard to make rules for these kids

The first two years in school have been used for the slow construction of a foundation. Now Clyde starts to teach at full force. Sometimes I feel that he is too effective. There must be a limit to the children's ability to learn.

In the morning we sing in sign language "Hello, friend." So far it's been expressionless and mechanical singing, imitating Clyde without the whole body following. I have seen the same kind of mechanical signing back home in Finland in sign choir performances that haven't been practiced enough. "Hello, friend" is being practiced every morning—we'll see if the children will adopt something of Clyde's fluid performance. His signs are not separate, but are connected fluently to each other like different notes in the melody of a song.

Bible study has been accepted into the schedules of all classes. "Wouldn't ethics be a better subject?" a friend of Clyde's asks. Though Clyde is not at all religious, Bible study seems to him more suitable than ethics. In St. Lucia people go to church a lot. "Believe in Him" and "God Protects" are painted on the buses. A crucifix hangs beside the bus driver; in all homes there are pictures of Jesus. Even at work people have a Bible near them.

For these reasons, children can't be completely ignorant of religion. Kenneth signs a devil with horns and points to the floor, then upwards—do I believe that there is a Devil and a God?

"Yes, I do," I say seriously.

Now Clyde teaches what sin is.

He draws on the board: a liquor bottle, cigarettes, bad books. They are the everyday sins. God doesn't like people to smoke, drink, or read bad books.

How about Clyde himself? I imagine Clyde takes a drink or two sometimes, so is he sinful? But Clyde doesn't answer the question. He is teaching now how one *should* live; maybe he doesn't care about being sinless.

"God loves good boys. God loves good girls. God loves good people."

The children copy sentences from the board into their notebooks. Surely they know God exists; He is somewhere up there, that's where the arrow is pointing to. But for them "God" and "good" are entwined into one and the same, there's only a difference of one letter between the words. God is good.

Sad and *happy.*

Thin and *thick.*

Look at the pictures: this person with the corners of his mouth turned down is sad, and this one who is smiling is happy. To express them one doesn't really need any signs; you can show happiness or sadness with your body.

S-a-d, a nice, short word to fingerspell and remember.

The children have to learn the concept and the English word and its American sign; they learn at the same time to write a word and to spell it in the hand alphabet.

The walls fill up fast with pictures and texts. The pictures of the sad and happy faces with their texts are left on the wall so they'll be in front of the children's eyes even when the faces aren't being taught. The children will remember only those words that have been repeated often enough during the lessons. Although the names of colors have been taught for two years, and now the colors and their names are on the wall for everybody to see, there's not one child, even among the most advanced group, who can remember all the colors, their signs, and their fingerspelling.

Clyde is satisfied. The room starts to look like a classroom where they have worked diligently. He hammers, saws, letters, draws. I letter, cut out pictures, glue, keep boxes in order.

"It must be tidy," Clyde says. But after a while when schoolwork is in full operation, the boxes will be all messed up because there won't be enough time to keep them in order. Religion, news as before—now the board is bigger, so more goes on it—grammar, new words, lunch, reading, math, biology, crafts, art. The days aren't long enough, and most days we're behind schedule. After cleaning up, we have a meeting. No, there's no time to keep everything in prime condition.

Every morning I go with bucket in hand to the neighboring kindergarten that's run by the Red Cross. The Canadian society that supports the kindergarten has sent us a big bag of milk powder, and the Red Cross stores the bag for us. We have visitors once in a while who want to help when they get back home, so they send something to the school. This milk powder is one of the finest ideas for helping, because what can minds learn when bodies get too little protein, and how can you speak with a toothless mouth? Now we can furnish some building material for children's teeth, bones, and brains.

The children are in school for a long day. Some have a piece of cake as lunch, some juice in bottles, some have money that they use to buy candy from the woman sitting by the gate: sour, tamarin balls that have a lot of vitamin C but much more sugar, or coconut roasted with sugar. The others don't have lunch at all—they look on while the others are eating the little they have along. Now at least everybody will have the milk and cookies that are given out during the ten o'clock break.

The days are sunny and hot. The windows on all sides of the classroom, which are opened in the morning and closed after school, bring some cool air into the room. The doors to the park are open. The park, with its bright sunlight and cheerful sounds, is a different world from this shady room, silent to the children. Sometimes they can't resist peering out at what's happening in the park. If one starts looking outside, so do the others. A person who can't hear has to look around as much as possible, and one has to tell the others what's happening because the others might not have seen it. Victor gestures to the others and laughs—until everybody feels a hard vibration along the table top, when Clyde beats it angrily with his palm, fed up with signing when the children are not even looking at him.

"Do you want to go to school?"

The hands come up at once.

"Of course! What would we do if there were no school!"

"Okay, then we work. Whoever wants to play can go home."

"Go home" equals "stay home" in every pupil's vocabulary.

Nobody wants to go home. Only Gregory has had to stay home; he can't come to school any more.

People are always walking through the park. Women in colorful dresses, schoolchildren in uniforms; the ice cream man pushes his brightly painted cart and rings his bell. Under the tree there's a man picking up breadfruits and dropping them into his wheelbarrow; another man dozes on a bench. Between the school buildings is a nursery where an old bent woman works with a straw hat on and a pipe between her teeth.

Just as we begin to work, heads appear in the windows. We might as well be in a cage for people to stare at.

People walking through the park peep in curiously through the open doors. Sometimes we let them be—Clyde thinks that letting people stare is one way to let more people know that the school for the deaf exists and that there are deaf children. Sometimes curious people come in and ask questions. Clyde hands them a sheet of paper, but not all of them know how to write what they want to know, and they go away.

Some of them gesture toward Clyde and ask me, "Doesn't he speak?"

I don't know what I should tell them. How could I ever explain the whole story?

"No, he doesn't speak, because he's deaf," would not be the right answer at all. "Yes, he does speak," wouldn't satisfy them either, because they can see that Clyde doesn't speak, not in the way they expect; he only writes on the paper. Clyde can express himself perfectly in sign language, but he can't pronounce speech quite the same way hearing people do. I feel that this question belittles Clyde, especially when it's asked behind his back. I am not pleased with these uninvited gawkers and visitors.

Not all of them understand deafness; there are always those who don't. I don't know why some people grasp the truth instinctively, while others misunderstand.

Sometimes intruders are persistent. They come over the threshold, peering at what has been written on the board or in the notebooks. Although I tell them to go away, they hang around the door until I'm very cross.

During every lesson Clyde writes on the board and the children write in their notebooks. I wonder how long they can stand to copy texts they don't understand. Kenneth understands most of it, Alfonso nothing at all.

But even Alfonso writes in his notebook, nice handwriting even though all the letters are copied straight from the board by rote. Their form has not yet been shaped in Alfonso's memory so that he can recognize the letters when he sees them written in a slightly different way from the prototype on the blackboard.

Alfonso sits beside Kenneth. Contrary to my expectations, Kenneth doesn't tease Alfonso; rather, they seem to be equals. Kenneth doesn't tease others for their stupidity as much as he used to.

There are spider webs hanging from the classroom ceiling. The ceiling is old and rotten, soaked from the rains. Once in a while rotten pieces of wood fall on us. In the dusty closets are old bottles and trash; mice run around there at night. On the floor, on top of the rotten planks, are bent remains of linoleum that we stumble on. But the table is strong and high enough for writing, the chairs are unbroken, and there are more than enough of them. The blackboard is large and strongly made. In this old, rotting house where the wind lazily flaps through the hot air, it's cozy.

Our class is like a school in itself. The smaller children in the other building on the other side of the yard seem to be in another time and place. When Clyde's class finishes its school days, one paragraph in the history of the deaf in St. Lucia will end. The younger children have it much easier already. More and more often now, a child's hearing impairment is found early. The mothers get guidance. They get information about sign language and about the school for the deaf. The school is already becoming a center where hearing tests are done and guidance and advice are given.

Between two and three o'clock there's a moment when the children refuse to take in any more information. They are limp and sleepy, sprawling against the table. They don't want to look at what I explain, although I try to tap one on the shoulder, or turn another's head by the chin. For many hours they've looked at us as we've taught, and copied words from the board into their notebooks. Can't it be time to finish and go home?

"Stop!" Finally Clyde hits the side of his palm on the other palm. Now the school day is over, but before we leave, we clean the classroom. Kenneth: close the windows. Joseph: pick up the papers from the floor. Victor: empty the waste basket. Theresa: sweep the floor. Valerie: wipe the board. Filipa: do the dusting. Alfonso: sweep the stairs.

Each week the tasks rotate, and of course everybody makes sure that they do only their part of the job and not one bit more.

"Home!" The fingers converge on the cheek and fly out from it—toward town or mountains or banana plantations.

Most of them have a long walk in the hot afternoon sun, with their heads full of knowledge and their stomachs empty, their shoe soles broken, their toes or teeth hurting. But how carefree and happy they look when they leave.

More often the youngsters stay in town after school. They want to spend a couple of hours together before they spread out, back to their homes. They'd surely like to be together even longer, but they always have to think of the sunset—darkness arrives all of a sudden at six or seven o'clock. It's quite dreadful to tramp home in the pitch dark, although it's a lot cooler then. 🐾

NOT TOO MUCH
OF ANYTHING

The blaze of the sun feels as heavy as a hundred-pound box on the top of my head. There seems to be a band around my head also, pressing even harder than the weight of the blazing sun. During lunch hour I dash into town to search for materials for crafts and other things we need at school. Clyde has made me the supplier of his kingdom, and he would like to have everything ready as soon as possible.

The palms are standing still. We wait for a small breeze to dry the sweat from our foreheads, but the wind has completely calmed down. Even in the evenings we perspire as we eat dinner on the balcony. If I go to the beach in pursuit of a cool breeze, the pinching of the sandflies is even worse than the heat.

And I don't have much time to go to the beach. Instead I run mindlessly all over town, to school, to the bus, dragging the grocery bag, with Alfonso following.

Until one day I feel the band pressing around my head from early morning until nightfall. I don't have the energy to go anywhere; I have to give in.

"I did warn you that you shouldn't start working full time, especially in this climate. But no, you have to try out everything before you believe it. It's my work that's the most important job over here, and I can't take care of anything if you're worn out," Jukka says angrily.

I would have had the energy to go on if it weren't so hot and if we didn't have Alfonso with us. Without him, my teaching would end at three o'clock, when school ends.

Sometimes I think that Jukka knows my energy resources better than I do myself. It's hard for me to admit to myself that I can't do everything I want to.

But inside myself, when I take a close look at it, I know that what has con
sumed my energy is my attempt to follow what people are saying, what they've
been saying for many years. In fact, I've been staring at people's lips with such
concentration that sometimes I forget to breathe. That's when I tire the most—
from lack of oxygen!

"You rest now," Jukka says determinedly. "Not until you have rested
enough can we start talking about working at the school again, and then only
from midday on. I can't handle things if you're tired and tense all the time—
nothing will get done around the house. Besides, it's my job that we're here for."

Jukka is really angry. Naturally he's always worried about my health; he
wants to see me brisk and well-rested. Not too much sun, not too much of anything. There must be a change in the order of my life; I realize it myself.

"Too much rest isn't good either," I say to Jukka. And although my teaching
is unpaid, I have to have some kind of work. I can't just stay at home. I'm not surprised at those women who fall into drinking over here—they don't have anything else to do.

I send a note for Clyde with Alfonso: I don't feel well; I'll rest at home for
the time being.

My father is worried because I'm so tired. He doesn't suffer much from the
heat, but then he was a tough sauna-goer when he was young. I remember how he
used to shout on the benches in the sauna: "Aijai! How it burns, burns!" and then
he'd throw more water on the hot stones.

After a time I didn't hear stories from my father any more; he'd already left
for the co-op butcher shop at five o'clock in the morning. In the evening he got
home tired and often drunk. I understood that my father's drinking was due to
the war and to hard work. I've always known that I was a dear daughter to my
father and that he has probably understood me better than anyone else, although
he has hardly ever said anything, and then only: "Dear Raija, I wonder how you
will get by in the world with that soft nature of yours."

Now, here on the island, as we sit for hours on the balcony conversing, we
grow closer. Father drinks coffee, one cup after another, and teases Victoria by
saying all kinds of funny things in Finnish. Sometimes I fetch some brown East
Indies rum for my father from the cupboard.

Father has finally found a style of speaking that enables me to understand him easily: slowly enough, with clear but not too exaggerated mouth movements, keeping the words apart. I should have explained this to him much earlier and not just waited for him to figure it out by himself.

When father's five-week vacation on the island is over, he's almost as tanned as he had hoped to be. We pack the shells and coral he collected from the shore, arrange guidance at Heathrow Airport for changing planes. It seems as if there's always somebody coming or going over the Atlantic.

MY LADY'S MAID, VICTORIA

crisis

Victoria is a good maid in her own way, but if she could, she would choose only to cook. She puts the whole day into cooking, and the results are good. We get delicious dinners which, according to St. Lucia custom, consist of many courses. Not until now have I really gotten to know the cuisine of the island—Victoria makes casseroles from the breadfruit and sweet potatoes, fries plantains, crisps battered christophene or green papaya in the oven.

You don't need to tell Victoria what should be done. She discovers everything herself, except what needs cleaning up.

"While you're at the beach I'll clean the *whole* house," Victoria says on Saturdays, spreading her arms dramatically.

In the beginning I believed her, but when we come back from the beach, after Victoria has gone home, the floors are full of scraps, and spiderwebs are still hanging from the same ceiling that Victoria was pointing at so energetically. The webs aren't really a sign that the house hasn't been cleaned for weeks. There are many spiders, and they spin more webs in a day than spiders in Finland do in a year.

The only accomplishment that Victoria has managed during the day are the four grapefruit halves on a dish decorated with red cocktail cherries, and the salad of green bananas and canned meat.

When I tell Victoria on Monday that the house wasn't clean on Saturday, she rolls her eyes in surprise and says: "Is that true?"

"Yes, the floor was full of scraps."

"Wasn't the kitchen floor clean?"

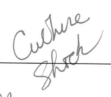

Well, yes, that was clean. Last thing before leaving for home, Victoria always sweeps the trash out straight through the door.

I understand that according to Victoria's sense of cleanliness, the house was already clean to start with. She had promised to clean the house, but because it was already clean, why do work for no reason?

Now that I'm home every day, Victoria wants to be my lady's maid. She is always there to zip my zipper; she fixes the rubber band in the showercap and fetches shoes for me—in Victoria's opinion a fine lady never walks around barefoot, not even at home. I like to go barefoot, now that I know that it's not at all dangerous. But here comes Victoria following me with the shoes!

"Your shoes, Madame! You have to be careful and keep tight to your husband. He is nice looking. There are so few men on the island. The women on the island, even at home, are tip-top."

Yes, there are women wishing for Jukka's company! If he looks at a girl a bit longer than a second, the girl asks at once: "You like me?"

I wonder if it's also for keeping my husband for myself that Victoria thinks that my underwear should be black. But I like white better. When I am on my way out to buy a petticoat, Victoria says: "Black! Madame, let me buy you a black petticoat!"

"No, I will find it myself."

"But I *like* black underwear," Victoria says.

That's fine with me, just so long as *I* don't need to wear black underwear.

Victoria is one of those people I always seem to run into—the ones who think that the make-up or dentist or whatever I use is not good enough, I should wear or buy the same thing they do. And what's worse, they think I should also *do* everything that they do: run ten kilometers every evening or bake three hundred cookies for Christmas or take up yoga or Spanish as a hobby.

A doubt starts creeping into my mind that perhaps Victoria is too strong a package for me. I believe that I can handle Victoria, but for some reason I often have the impression that she has gulled me.

"Victoria, you came very late today. It's already eleven."

"Oh, Madame, there was so much folk at the market, I had to wind in and out like this."

Victoria shows me visually how she has wound in and out in the crowd at

— 160 —

the market. And besides that, she has searched for the best possible sweet potatoes and yams for the cheapest possible price. Victoria explains exactly how much everything has cost. They are cheap, I have to admit. I would have to pay much more for the same thing. But I'm sure that a small commission is included for Victoria herself.

Or when I tell Victoria that she can take home only the food that I've reserved for her on the kitchen table, she spreads her arms piously:

"I don't take anything; I go to church every Sunday."

To make that very obvious, Victoria has a Bible with her at work. Fine, fine, but then what about the fried plantains and chicken legs that she slides into the vegetable closet on the sly to take home later? Out of six plantains, three arrive fried on the table; the rest go into Victoria's storage.

"This is my lunch I didn't have," Victoria explains. Or: "Madame, I took some macaroni and one grapefruit yesterday."

This is okay in Victoria's opinion because she asks for permission—afterwards. Our understanding differs so completely that agreement is impossible. Zenia always understood what was hers, and she never took anything home except what I had reserved for her. But Victoria is everything Zenia is not. Victoria is polite and considerate. She's happy, singing in the kitchen and smiling as she cuts vegetables. Victoria's most common word is "like," to like something.

"I am so *happy* that you're on the island." She sings and smiles also as she irons: "I *like* ironing!"

When I tell her that we're going to have dinner guests, she shouts: "I'll do overtime. I *like* to work late!"

I guess I have exactly the kind of maid I've always wanted!

An especially good side to Victoria is her ability to communicate with me. She knows how she should talk to me: slowly, clearly, and by moving the lips but not exaggerating. Victoria stands in front of me, looks at me closely, and then speaks. Usually I understand what she says, and I learn many new words, such as "flavor" instead of "taste" when one means the taste of food.

F-l-e-i-v-o-r, Victoria says slowly.

I wonder first what "sebntiin" or "sebnti" means, but then I understand that's how "seventeen" and "seventy" are pronounced. And from then on I understand all the sevens in prices at the marketplace. The spoken language is best learned by speaking. A deaf child doesn't learn the language of the environment properly because he can't hear it being spoken. After almost a year on the island I don't speak English any better than I did when we arrived. I have read piles of English books; I have proceeded from easier texts into more difficult ones, and there are a lot of words in my mind, but how on earth are they pronounced? It's hard to use words in your speech when you haven't heard them, but have only seen them in books.

Joppe tries to correct my pronunciation. He has the ability to pronounce well. When he was small, he spoke to me extremely clearly, and it was very easy for me to understand what he said.

"Don't say 'piiil' for 'people.' It's like 'pupil.' Say 'piipl.' Or "It's 'dzuus,' not 'juus.'"

But how in the world do I distinguish all the different sounds so that I know when I say them right?

"Show me where your tongue is when you say 'mother'."

Joppe lifts his chin. Under the lamp in bright light I try to see where his tongue is during that strange sound.

"Now say 'think'."

Well, what's the difference between them? The sounds look alike.

How about when some lady sighs, "I'm dying for a cup of tea."

I could never thrust myself onto a sofa and sign naturally, "I'm dying for a cup of coffee!"

I have seen the idiom in a book, but I've never heard it being used in real life, and that's a completely different matter.

Now Victoria brings some real life into my English.

At the end of September it's Joppe's birthday. Victoria spends the entire day making the cake. She beats the butter long and earnestly, each egg just as long— separately. She pours in the vanilla and the almond essence without which no cakes are made on the island. She tastes and pours again until there's just the right shade of flavor.

And now the careful baking. It's no wonder that the cake will be well baked and even, not higher anywhere, not split anywhere. I've never seen such a cake!

Victoria makes the icing out of powdered sugar, lime peel, and cherries. Before she goes home she goes out and fetches colorful branches from bushes that look like flowers and spreads them all over the house. She puts them in old coffee cans and wraps napkins around them, because I haven't bought vases, and not much else either. There's no point in purchasing everything for a temporary stay.

In the evening the birthday guests come: Cornell and Mary Charles and their children Liza, Ian, and David. Mary is from California; she is a nurse and specializes in therapy for mentally disturbed patients. She has become the island's expert on disabled people. To my surprise, she doesn't think she knows all the issues concerning deafness, but often asks me for my opinion.

Liza speaks to me slowly, with clear mouth movements. In the Charles's company I never feel the need to repress aggression. They are at the most positive end of the scale from "understanding" to "not understanding."

JERI FLIES TO
THE CARIBBEAN

Jeri is a noteworthy dog. He's a Rottweiler, the son of Attalos Assi and Osman of Katajisto. He has had good training from the time he was ten months old. When he was two years old, he earned the required points in the obedience test and became tax-free. He became a member of the rescue organization that is always preparing for something new: to search for people trapped in ruins, to follow traces of people lost in forests. We went with Jeri to training camps and contests. In the winter he drew a sleigh with a 66-pound sandbag for weight; Jukka skied behind him, holding onto the reins.

We also went with Jeri to shows, where he already had won a certificate. Of course we were awfully proud. The second time Jeri won, he couldn't get a certificate because at that time he didn't have obedience points. At the next show Jeri won second prize in the open category, but didn't make it to the winners' category and so was not even close to the certificate. We looked unbelieving at the small blue ribbon Jeri received. We were close to crying and were very angry at the woman judge. Jeri has perfect form, his body is excellent—but from his mother he has inherited a narrow head, which some judges don't like, while others don't consider it a fault at all.

We got tired of the whole business. And we couldn't completely commit ourselves to this strange world that took all our weekends.

Jeri is also a widely traveled dog. At the age of six months he flew with us to Lapland, guarded a wilderness hut, and slept one night in the bridal suite of the Hotel Pohjanhovi and two nights at Ounasvaara. The wall-to-wall carpets were in danger, but nobody on the hotel staff said anything.

Later on Jeri served as boat dog in our boat. He visited the archipelago of Turku and the Åland Islands. He grasped well that he was looking after our safety, overnight at busy boat harbors. He got his strength back by sleeping deeply during sea voyages. He always had a life jacket on when on the boat. People laughed when they saw Jeri sitting in the bow, looking important with his life jacket on.

Jeri has also sailed through the Saimaa Canal. He got permission to come back from the Soviet Union's side of the border without quarantine by promising that he would not put his paws on Soviet soil. It was hard to keep that promise, but it was kept.

And now Jeri is taking the long journey west to the island!

I start to worry. Suppose Jeri can't take this warm climate? He's big and black. He'll get worms and illnesses. He's used to sleeping on the bed and the sofa—what if he gets fleas over here, as all dogs do? What if Victoria is afraid of Jeri? All islanders are afraid of dogs, especially big, fierce-looking ones. I'm sure to be faced with a search for a new maid. And of course I'll need to make sure that Alfonso won't act carelessly with Jeri.

But how I wait for Jeri! I dream about how he jumps out of the car, sees Joppe and me, dashes up the stairs, wags his tail, jumps up and licks us, wild with joy after the long separation.

Then another awful image creeps into my mind. What if Jeri won't let himself be put into the plane for the journey? And even worse: Jeri will be forgotten, won't be put into the second plane in London but will be left in the big airport for days.

I'm not the only dog-lover in our family. Letters, telexes, and telephone calls are sent to Finland and London. Where Jeri is concerned, expense is not spared, but those expenses get my blessing.

On Sunday afternoon when Jeri, according to our calculations, should be in London, we are overwhelmed by a horrible feeling that he will be abandoned at Heathrow Airport. This frightening thought makes us drive to town. Jukka sends a telex: "Our best friend is coming to St. Lucia on flight BA. . . . We would be very grateful if you could take care that he is put on the right plane."

The next day a telex arrives from British Airways in London: "Your pal Jeri is on the plane." English friendliness at its best. Jukka leaves to meet him at Hewanorra. I sit with Joppe and Alfonso on the balcony and wait.

We can see one plane after another landing at Vigie Airport, but no sign of Jukka and Jeri. It gets dark; we turn on the lights and light the mosquito coils. The dinner gets cold; insects are having a party on the dishes.

"I wonder when they will get here," Joppe says once in a while.

Alfonso just sits and looks around. After he has come home from school and taken a swim on the shore, he doesn't know what else to do. For hours he just sits and watches. Now he is looking at two colorless gecko lizards that always appear on the ceiling planks above the balcony. They lie in wait for the insects flapping around. Open a mouth: Snap! One bite of the evening meal goes into the stomach.

It's nine-thirty in the evening when the car finally drives into the yard. An angry, tired, and dirty Jukka climbs out of the car first, and after him a huge dog, so black he can hardly be seen in the tropical darkness. With Joppe, I look in astonishment at the clumsy lump of black fur, with his big head on his short, fat neck.

Jeri is so huge! We have completely forgotten that—in only a year.

Is it Jeri standing there? But he doesn't come to greet us with his tail wagging. He doesn't even notice us. He's wet from saliva, he's dirty; his tongue is hanging out. He stumbles around in the house as if he's blind.

Joppe, Alfonso, and I run up and down the kitchen stairs with warm water, shampoo, towels, brushes, paw cream.

With his usual thoroughness, Jukka washes Jeri with warm water and foamy shampoo for over an hour. Jukka is angry. The plane was late because of engine trouble. Jeri had been sweating in the furnace-hot Antigua airport for three hours, then had to spend another hour and a half at Hewanorra because customs refused to handle his papers or even let him out.

"It might be the case that we don't even have time today," they said.

On the island a dog's position is different from that back home in Finland. Island dogs look shaggy, not cared for at all, hungry, full of fleas. People don't understand that one well-treated dog is a better guard for the house than a bunch of mistreated ones.

The customs official can't guess that there's a special dog in the box. Jukka blows up, and they finally look at Jeri's papers and open the box.

When the box is opened, a huge black creature dashes, muddleheaded, out of the box. Everyone flees in terror against the walls. Some kind of wild beast has been let loose! But on Jukka's command, the beast sits down, well-behaved.

I laugh. I would have loved to have seen the men's expressions when Jeri dashed out of his prison!

Washed clean, Jeri gets some light food. He tries to sleep, but everything is too strange. Jeri is now on St. Lucia. It's hard to believe.

After a couple of days Jeri recovers from the strain of the trip. He begins to get familiar with the strange new smells and sounds around him. He wonders at the green lizards that catch insects on the walls and floors, at small frogs that jump out from under the kitchen door, at big cockroaches that dash to and fro on the walls, swiveling their antennas. At first he barks all night long because the night is filled with the endless barking and howling of other dogs, sometimes escalating to turmoil when the males fight. But soon Jeri gets used to it. He remembers Joppe and me and the old life. He starts to listen, with tilted head, to what he is told, and he understands everything.

When Alfonso comes upstairs in the morning, he doesn't waver for a moment, although of course Jeri barks and shoots off toward him. Maybe Alfonso doesn't understand Jeri's threatening tone of voice because he doesn't hear it. Because Alfonso shows no fear, Jeri stops trying to terrify him. I had forgotten Alfonso's close connection with Nature. Of course, like all the other islanders, he's afraid of dogs, but he can see that Jeri is not just any common barker who runs away when he sees a stick.

Alfonso spreads his arms and tells me that he flew during the night! He has floated in the air around the whole globe and seen the North Pole under him. The North Pole! This must be the first time Alfonso has been off the island even in his sleep. All the books and magazines whose pictures he has studied, my stories about the globe, about the sun and the moon and their movements finally have got organized in his thoughts. Maybe Jeri's popping up from somewhere far away has helped this development a bit.

I explain for Alfonso that it was a dream, that he was sleeping in his own bed and saw images, like movies. Imagination and reality get mixed up in Alfonso's consciousness, and his vocabulary doesn't include the word "dream" yet.

Victoria isn't afraid of Jeri either, but all the others are afraid, more or less. And that's good. This way our house won't be visited on illegal business too easily. I feel safe again: I hear Jeri's hollow barking, but not the quiet step of somebody entering. Jeri lets me know if somebody is coming near the house. I can distinguish from his voice who or what is approaching. Jeri also knows how to communicate with me using facial expressions. He comes to the door and looks at me happily: "Father comes," his expression says. Then there's "Where's my dinner?", the expression he uses to tell me that I haven't fed him and it's past dinnertime. Who says that communication is only speaking, only for humans?

DINNER ON A
BANANA BOAT

I take along an extra hearing aid battery in my evening bag—I won't go anywhere without that, because if I do, the old battery will lose power after half an hour, like film ending in a camera at the worst possible moment.

The evening bag is moldy, and I can tell from that that we haven't been anywhere for a long time. And I also notice that I haven't checked and ventilated the closets for a long while. I always take Jukka's thick suits and overcoat outside when the weather is dry and sunny, but lately it's been hot and wet and pouring rain. During the rainy season clothes and mattresses smell of mold all the time, the pages of books are curled, drawers go stale.

Besides weariness from the heat, I'm in good spirits. I realize that I've charged my batteries at home for a long time. I have not yet, however, reached the point where every visit, every communication situation is not an ordeal demanding effort to cope with.

I often wonder what Jukka thinks when he says many times during an evening: "My wife is deaf." I still cling to Jukka too much, although he sometimes shakes me off, forces me to get along alone, and I've noticed that it's easier if I handle things myself. People make better contact with me. If they can't use Jukka as an interpreter but have to find a way, they do, if they try hard enough. Surprisingly, many people do have that kind of will. There are people here who have traveled all over the world, couples from completely different corners of the world from one other. Perhaps people who have seen the world are not surprised at anything. Maybe I've already started to get my priorities straight.

After pondering for a while, I put the gilded pen Jukka has given me and a small note pad in my bag. I could try these out, to see if they help. What did that book say that I borrowed from Clyde? That it is my responsibility to inform every new group of people I meet: "People can be embarrassed because they don't know how to communicate with a hearing-impaired person." But the other side of the coin is that information doesn't always get through. I wonder if I have informed people correctly and bravely enough? Perhaps not. Mentioning a hearing impairment usually causes confusion. This goes away when people get to know me better. Then they forget that there are any problems at all and start talking to me a lot.

Once I was dancing with a stranger. He told me something, although people here don't usually talk while dancing.

"Sorry, I don't hear; I have lost my hearing."

At that moment, the boy's dancing started to be uncertain, although we had danced well before.

"I do hear the rhythm of the music with my hearing aid," I told the boy.

And then we resumed dancing skillfully. Yes, people can't know what I hear and what I don't, so I have to remember my responsibilities.

The book says that you have to be happy and friendly and should not make an issue of the fact that you don't hear. Well, I have smiled for hours in my life without knowing what was going on, so as the years have passed, my smile has grown chilly. But I can find a way to start smiling again.

We're on our way to a dinner party on the "Geestland" banana boat.

They tell me that it wasn't too long ago that the banana loads swung from the tops of women's heads in baskets to the boat: an unbroken chain of women with heavy baskets on their heads, diligent as ants. I can imagine it easily, because the women on the island carry everything on their heads. They have erect posture and walk nimbly.

From the captain's salon there opens up a familiar view—the peaked bow of the boat, cranes lifting loads into the gaping holds below, masts and lights, mastlights. After the boat goes out to sea, the holds will be closed, the deck deserted; the sharp bow will sink down and rise up again.

How many times I have stared at this sight from Jukka's cabin or from the command deck during his watch. I still love boats and the sea, but living as a wife of a sailor is like the rising and falling of the boat's bow. On the downswing it was sometimes very difficult—waiting, often for months at a time; having responsibility for children and household business. I have sympathy for sailors. They are as much misunderstood as any other group with which people are unfamiliar.

We shake hands with everybody, as is the custom in our country. Others shake hands only if they have not met before and not always even then. Sometimes someone gives a kiss on the cheek; it feels good, and sometimes when an older lady offers her cheek I know what to do.

Communication flows as easily as water. Jukka interprets quick as lightning; I answer, speaking as much as possible. I try to pronounce as clearly as possible and if my words aren't clear enough, Jukka helps out, skillfully and without fuss. An excellent performance!

Later I get separated from Jukka. I'm afraid for a moment when people come close to me. I fear that someone will start a discussion, and what do I do then? But when a man beside me starts chatting, I drag out my pen and paper determinedly. And it's worth it. The man is Mr. Twyford, who studies bananas—how they grow best, how they can best be packed, and so on.

It's not hard for me to be interested, because the banana tree is one of the small wonders of the world. I can see in our own garden how the banana tree dries out; beside it, new leaves start emerging, all curled up, and soon there's a new tree in its place with a few white flowers. The fruit develops inside a violet funnel. I have learned that there are no seeds in the banana plant, but that the tree propagates from its root. I've never heard of that before.

I feel that I've made contact with this banana researcher.

While we're having dinner, the captain of the ship comes up to me and asks if the meal is good. I answer by showing him the thumb-and-forefinger circle for "excellent," a sign that even hearing people use. The captain laughs and makes the same sign. One sign, and the contact is better than if I had said, "Thank you, this cake is excellent."

I get the feeling that I've crossed a threshold. I don't know how it happened and if it really happened during that evening, but I'm not suffering strain from people any more. Suddenly it's as if some barrier had vanished from between me and hearing people. But still I feel, even more clearly than before, that I never can belong to their world; it's impossible. I'll always hang in between the two worlds. But maybe I'll gradually learn to hang right, to find the footpath.

On our way back home Jukka teases me about the captain being so considerate. He took me by the hand to get my dessert; he offered me chocolate.

"I guess he liked you!"

It's Jukka's way to lift my self-confidence. 🐚

ROASTING DAYS

It's not very nice to stay at home. I feel that I'm being lazy when somebody else bustles about in my kitchen and does the work I'm used to doing, the work that filled my days back home. Living here on the island is interesting, but not rich in the same way as at home. Here you have to find something to do, whereas there you had to find time for everything that had to be done.

It feels particularly sad to be on the outside of what's happening at school. I get information about that only through Alfonso or, to be more precise, I guess from Alfonso's stories what has happened each day. But the sun still is too smothering. During the day I can't even sit on the balcony; in spite of the shade from the lianas, the sunshine exhausts me. The town is hot as a furnace in the afternoons. They say that it hasn't been this hot for decades. People can't sleep at night in town because the concrete walls store the heat of the sun during the day and glow during the night like ovens. Everybody would like to escape, to go up near the volcano in the mountains where the air is always cool and fresh, the healthiest on the island. The sulfur smells bad up there, but maybe it does you good.

But somehow there's always exceptional weather on the island. The climate seems to follow a pattern in long cycles: twenty years from now, the weather will again be similar to today's.

Joppe comes home from school in the afternoons at two-thirty, glowing red and sweaty, even though the school is only a stone's throw away. He asks Victoria for lime juice with a lot of ice and rolls filled with butter and ham. Victoria serves Joppe willingly, and he knows how to use this willingness.

He sits down in a chair, puts a record on, and concentrates on his eating and reading. He doesn't say anything to me. The only thing he says the whole afternoon is "I'll go swimming," when he's on his way to the beach with a towel on his shoulder. I am allowed neither to watch over him nor to wave.

Those times seem so long ago when the most important moment of the day was when Joppe came home from school and told me everything that had happened.

But there's still a small boy in Alfonso. He doesn't get home until four or five o'clock, because he has to walk three miles, and most days he idles along in town before coming home. He watches the boats in the harbor, men playing dominoes on the pavements, fishing boats near where he sold paper before. Sometimes I wonder if he misses that colorful life in the town and the mountains, the village life that he's used to. Our house is in a very quiet area. There's nothing happening in the evenings. There's nothing but darkness, sparks of fireflies, and lights from neighboring houses. Not a single person is sitting on stairs or dancing in dusky streets.

As soon as Alfonso gets home he looks for me and tells me vividly what has happened during the day. I "listen," interpreting the message the whole time in my mind, remembering always that he might have completely misunderstood the whole matter or I might misunderstand what he's telling me. If we both misunderstand, the whole message is lost.

I do know, however, that there's a new girl in the class whose name starts with an M and that a doctor has visited the school and examined all the children, even the babies. He has examined the heart, ears, and lungs.

"You healthy?"

"Yes," Alfonso nods.

I think that his heart and lungs may be okay, but I've often thought of taking him to the doctor to find out what his health is really like. Does he have anemia? Is his stomach all right?

As Alfonso talks to me, I observe how his language is developing. It amuses me to see all the new signs he's learned at school, mixed in with his own gestures. Sometimes it's as if a hearing person would include some complicated high-culture word in an everyday discussion.

But Alfonso and I gradually have more and more common language. Sometimes when all the circumstances are favorable and we both are at our best, our ways of thinking meet, and a contact is born. It surprises me that when we do have a good mutal understanding, that's when Alfonso becomes arrogant, and bang! All that's good is gone. I have to treat the boy more coolly again. I just can't understand it.

Besides his own signs and the ones he's learned in school, Alfonso uses all kinds of vague gestures that I have difficulty understanding. All that he doesn't quite know how to "say" is expressed in squares, triangles, and circles. He might come and ask me for a square.

What? I don't understand. He stands at the door with an inquiring, questioning look. He shows the square again and again, and his laugh tells me that I'm nuts when I don't understand. And soon he learns the sign for "nuts." You can't avoid learning it in school, because it's the most common scolding word among the children.

It's not easy to take it calmly when you're called nuts!

"Listen to me. Many things are squares."

I show him things in the kitchen for which one could use that sign. Alfonso understands and makes a gesture describing washing, rubbing his fists together as if washing something.

I see! You mean washing powder! I give him the detergent box from the closet. But the next time the square means a napkin or a piece of toast! And the more precise formulation doesn't come until he's told me that I'm dumb.

When I think more carefully about it, these squares and circles and other shapes are things that Alfonso doesn't know any gesture or sign for. They haven't been brought up in our discussions; they're things that didn't exist in Alfonso's earlier life. There were no napkins or toast, and maybe no washing powder either. How could he know how to express the idea? I solve the problem by teaching Alfonso to make a precise formulation of the forms; a square plus a washing gesture means the detergent box.

It's really quite natural to expect the other person to understand the idea that's so clear in your own mind.

I also have to interpret the words Alfonso spells out every afternoon. He wants to show me what he has learned. He moves his fingers, forms letters with them, and then puts a forefinger to his pursed lips.

"Who?" I have given up hoping that he will distinguish "what" from "who," because the other children don't do that either.

Sometimes—rarely—the letters formed by the fingers really are words, often after a little correction.

"WOC," Alfonso fingerspells proudly.

"Who?"

No, that's not quite right.

He ponders for a moment.

"COW," his fingers tell me.

"Cow, right. Good. It's a cow." I show the sign for a cow, the fingers forming horns on the forehead.

And happily Alfonso tries another word.

"PIG."

"Pig. Good!"

Slowly and painfully he learns words, maybe one per month.

Alfonso doesn't get depressed, even when the fingerspelled letter combination isn't a word and doesn't mean anything. He doesn't seem to have any sense of ignorance and failure; he knows everything, he can do everything! And I'm too tactful to tell anybody straight to his face that he doesn't know anything. Although Alfonso calls me dumb, I won't call him that.

And sometimes I don't feel very wise. I'm constantly fumbling around in deep darkness, trying out various procedures to determine which works best in teaching him.

One afternoon Alfonso has company with him.

I am resting in the bedroom, where it's a few degrees cooler than on the sunny side in the afternoon.

He comes to me proudly makes a J-letter on his forehead.

Surprised, I go to the balcony, and Joseph is sitting there, sweating.

"Joseph! How are you, Joseph?"

Every day, every child is asked individually, "How are you?" and everybody answers, "I am fine," but Joseph doesn't know how to put his learning to use outside the classroom.

"Fine?" I answer for Joseph.

I get juice and coconut cake for the boys, and Alfonso is playing host. He shows the books and things in the living room proudly, as if our home were his home, too, and that's what I've been hoping for—that he would consider this his home, that we could adapt on both sides. He points to photos as if to show off his own family members, and that's also quite all right; we are his family if he wants it that way. It all depends on how he understands the whole matter and on how I can express these things to him. And it depends on a lot of other things, too, things that I can't get a handle on right now.

But now, right now, Alfonso is a part of our family, and our house is his home.

YESTERDAY, TODAY, TOMORROW

Sometimes when Alfonso comes up from the beach he yells to let us know that he's home. His voice is hollow and rough. I wonder how he figured out that he has a voice he can draw attention with.

"Tell that boy not to yell when he comes from the beach," Jukka says.

I explain this to Alfonso.

One day when he's explaining something and signing, he suddenly pronounces clearly: "Biig!" The "i" is long as the sign and as big as the thing he's describing.

The children in school know how to say short, simple words or the first syllables of words without any teaching, like "fa-fa-fa." They see the mouth-movement pattern of the word many times, copy it, and instinctively add sound to it. Of course it's impossible for me to distinguish how well they can pronounce it, but at least the lip pattern is right.

This must have happened to Alfonso, too. He copies the lip movements in words like "pen," "man," and "big," although there's not much difference in pronunciation of the letter "p," "m," and "b."

He tells expressively how the doctor has come to the school, how the students have visited a warship, how the class will take a trip to the Pitons. It's especially easy for me to follow the description of the warship, because I'm acquainted with so many boats. Everything is new and marvelous for Alfonso, and the description ends with a flapping of the hand. I wonder what that gesture actually means. For me it means "huh," as if a person who is hot is fanning his face with something. I must ask Clyde what it means. Alfonso seems to have learned it in school recently.

Alfonso also tells me that they are being taught to speak. He shows how the earphones are put on the ears, and then he puts his hand on the throat and utters sounds. Well, teaching speech is a bit late for these children now. If they were taught all day long, they would not learn to speak in the time they still have left in school. But we've received a fine "Auditory Training Unit" with earphones and amplifiers as a gift, and some eager volunteer has decided to teach the children to speak.

Often, even on Saturday mornings, Alfonso appears for breakfast with his school outfit on.

"No school today. Put your old clothes on. Tomorrow no school. After tomorrow Monday. On Monday to school."

Every evening Alfonso asks when he leaves with the mosquito coil in his hand to go downstairs to bed: "Tomorrow school?"

"Yes." I nod my fist, it's like a nodding head.

"Yes, tomorrow is a school day. And tomorrow-tomorrow and tomorrow-to-morrow-tomorrow. And tomorrow-tomorrow-tomorrow-tomorrow. Then no school, and we go swimming. We stay at home for two days. On Sunday you go to the movies. The next day is Monday, then again school."

I point to the calendar on Alfonso's wall.

"Look. Now is this day, today. This is 'tomorrow'." I show the whole row of numbers. "This is a week. And this whole page is a month." I show that soon the pages on the calendar will end. All the pages are a year. When all the pages are gone, a new year starts.

To my surprise Alfonso understands. He points to town.

Yes, that's when there will be sellers at the market!

Finally I get another calendar and take it to Alfonso's room.

"Look, now is today. I put a cross over the number. Tomorrow you open your eyes."

"You take a pen and do like this. And again when you wake up, you do the same thing. This red circle is Sunday. Then you don't have school. This other "S" is Saturday, no school then, either."

One evening Alfonso signs, "Finished?"

"What? What finished?"

"School finished," Alfonso signs.

Alfonso asks if there's school tomorrow. "Finished" in the children's language means something that has been done, which is finished, but it also means something that doesn't exist. They've enlarged the meaning of the word and the sign.

Or when Alfonso is going out the kitchen door and down the stairs to his room to bed, he remembers something. I think he's asking as much to make contact with me as to find out facts.

"Later?"

"What? What is 'Later?'"

"Later school?"

"Yes. You sleep first, then later school."

"Later" is used a lot at school, associated with the concept "finished." Alfonso couldn't help learning it. The children have also changed this sign. It should actually be the forefinger and thumb of the right hand turning on the left palm like clockhands, but the children rest only the thumb on the palm and let the other fingers swing forward and downward.

These time concepts are discussed every day, especially now that I have told Alfonso that Joppe and I will soon fly "fa-fa-fa."

"Man fly? Dog fly?"

"No, Man-Who-Carries-Briefcase stays here. Woman cooks and gives food to Alfonso. Raija and Joppe fly. Later Raija flies back (a plane coming back). Joppe does not fly back. Joppe stays fa-fa-fa school."

Alfonso looks satisfied. I don't know if he's satisfied because his fighting partner is staying fa-fa-fa school or because Raija will come back. But Alfonso is worried about the matter, and I have to explain to him many times that he will be taken care of; he won't be alone.

Yes, I have decided to visit Finland. I'll take Joppe, buy him winter clothes, arrange the boys' lives, and refresh myself. I have been on the island for a year, and sometimes I feel like going to a big, busy place instead. I need to meet people and talk to them. I have dreamed many times about going back and visiting my friends, one after another. I dream that I walk along, enjoying the town; I look at the beautiful, stylish things in the shop windows, sit in cafes and watch the life around me, and read books and magazines. I'm greedy from the bottom of my heart for what I've been without over here, for what I've been craving for the whole year.

Sometimes I feel that I won't have the energy to stay here, although most of the time I'm satisfied. In the beginning I was really happy and worry-free. I made a big fuss over the mold or the cockroaches for no reason—these were not real problems. The only real problem was Keke's and Joppe's adjustment, because they did have it hard.

Here, for the first time in my life, I could live just as I wanted. There was nobody telling me what I should do or should not do. There were no magazines with ads demanding that I should buy this and that, dress a certain way, use make-up like this. Nothing could make my home seem shabby. There were not always go-getting, top-notch, energetic people beside whom my own capacity seemed like zero. Well, there was Jukka of course, but I've always thought that Jukka needs his opposite at home.

After six months or so, the enchantment of the new environment began to fade, and in July I started missing Finland very much. How is it that a person feels instinctively that it's summer back home, without even thinking about it consciously? It's hard over here to imagine the weather back home; in January it felt very strange to think that it really is January now, and that they have snow and cold in Finland.

And the climate on the island, which is so wonderfully fresh and uplifting in the winter, has become even wetter, hotter, and heavier since May. Here the connection between spirit and weather, especially in regard to humidity, is much clearer than in Finland. Those friends back home who long for faraway countries think this is a wonderful sun island—a place where every day is like the most wonderful summer days in Finland. The reality is far from that!

culture shock   part of crisis

INCIDENT AT THE DENTAL CLINIC

For days Alfonso has had a sore tooth. The boy's teeth look very strong. The front teeth are yellower than those of most islanders, but they haven't any black spots. The molars also look good, with no visible holes. Only the first adult lower tooth on each side is completely broken and rotten.

I give him some aspirin, but something should be done about those teeth. They're "finished," as Valerie says of her teeth, which have almost all been pulled because of abscesses.

I ask Maureen to call the dental clinic and get an appointment for Alfonso. I go to the same clinic myself; it's supported by the American Adventist Church. For the locals it's quite an expensive clinic, but compared with Finnish prices it's very cheap.

We sit in the waiting room and look at a picture book that tells about Noah's Ark and the deluge. The story seems to interest Alfonso, and I tell him how Noah took two of each species in his ark, female and male. Surely the islanders can easily imagine the Deluge! They have those kinds of days every year during the rainy season in November.

The others in the waiting room look at our signing a bit, but they aren't as curious as people usually are. In a dentist's waiting room, who would be interested in anything else but the thought of having to sit in the torture chair! I don't understand why I dread going to the dentist even though the tooth is numbed before being drilled.

The receptionist calls us to the counter. I explain that I don't hear, that she must write for me. The boy is also deaf.

"You remember, I have been here before, but now I bring this boy; he has a couple of badly broken teeth."

The receptionist nods and gives the boy an examining look.

From earlier visits to the clinic I know that before examination and care you have to fill out a detailed form. I have pondered how I would fill it out, because I don't know anything about Alfonso.

His first name I know, but how about his last name, and birth date, not to mention all the illnesses he has had, and any allergies that the clinic needs to know about?

I really can't write anything but the name Roger and our address.

"You see," I explain to the receptionist, "we have taken the boy to live at our house; we take care of him, so he can go to the school. I've taught him in school. Unfortunately, even the school doesn't know his last name and birth date."

"Doesn't the boy himself know his last name?"

"No, he doesn't know. He knows only a couple of words of English; he can't read or write. I talk with him in sign language, but we are able to communicate only a little."

The receptionist looks at the boy, puzzled. She doesn't know what to do.

"I must have seen that boy before . . ."

The woman disappears into the dentist's office with the papers. After a while she comes back and puts pen and paper in front of Alfonso.

I look over his shoulder at what stands out on the paper: *ROGER*.

They are actually trying to lead him to write his name, last name and all! The situation is comic, and shows once again that people really don't know anything about deafness and its consequences!

Alfonso starts scribbling the name Roger. He copies it on the paper: both "Name" and "Roger"! Oh, God, he's been copying in school, what else could he think now but that he should copy again? He doesn't remember how to write his first name; it's not so long ago that he accepted the idea that he has a name at all.

The receptionist glances at me, even more puzzled.

I don't say anything, but in my mind I say, "You idiot! I told you that the boy doesn't know how to read or write and doesn't know his last name. That is the situation—down to the very letter."

Again the receptionist disappears into the doctor's office, and after a while, still embarrassed, she comes out and asks us in.

In the consulting room I begin to panic. I realize all of a sudden that I've taken the responsibility for what will happen to Alfonso. In a little while he could get a numbing needle in his gum, and soon after that he could have a tooth pulled that's badly abscessed and dangerous. Besides, I dread this consulting room, chair, and dentist even though I don't need to sit in the chair myself with my mouth wide open, feeling helpless.

I stand there rooted to the spot, but then I'm asked to go back to the waiting room. There I sit and wait until Alfonso comes out, pressing his cheek.

I ask the receptionist when we have to come back, because I don't think both of the teeth were taken out at the same time. But there won't be any next time! I don't quite understand, but I decide to leave it as it is. I guess the teeth were so badly broken that the clinic can't take them both out without knowing anything about the possible risks. I don't dare do anything about the matter before I know more about the boy. Anyway, what right do I have to have teeth extracted from a boy I picked up in the street?

For the first time I come to think of the legal aspects of this "picking up." It's surprising that even Jukka has not thought about this. How far does our responsibility for the boy reach?

But the problem is forgotten because in a couple of days Alfonso feels completely well. And the other tooth doesn't hurt any more, although I notice that the tooth that he said hurt most is still in its place, and a tooth was pulled out on the opposite side.

VICTORIA'S ASTRONAUT HELMET

One morning Victoria looks a bit strange. She has a new uniform on, and her hair is in waves that turn up at the ends. She does look stylish, but I liked her hair better as it was before: in small pigtails tied with rubber-band balls. Oh well, if I curl my hair with a perm, why shouldn't Victoria be allowed to straighten hers?

It took three hours and half of Victoria's weekly salary to straighten her hair. But she happily hums religious songs in the kitchen, takes dancing steps in between, and claps her hands. And in the afternoon she asks if she can take home butter and guava jam. She doesn't ask for herself, but for her children!

Victoria knows that children are my weak point—for whom would they not be? I give Victoria, or her children, a whole jar of guava jam. She made it herself, and there are still many jars in the fridge.

Victoria really is talented in so many ways. Even the uniform she's wearing shows that! First I gave her some material so that she could get a uniform made. But then she started asking if she could get another one, too. I understand that there have to be two uniforms, so that the second one can be washed. She doesn't have the kinds of dresses in her wardrobe that she can wear while she works in the kitchen. I give her money for the material. After a while she tells me shyly that the material she bought was enough for two uniforms. Could Madame pay for a seamstress to make two uniforms?

I give her the money, but I am angry, both because of my own stupidity and because of Victoria's games. The girl uses me. Although I tell her straight out what I'm thinking, she doesn't take me seriously. The worst I can do is to tell Jukka, because Victoria fears Jukka.

The next day Victoria comes to work with big pink rollers in her hair. The rollers are in her hair from morning til evening day after day, and I wonder when she takes them out, to show off the beautiful curls. I wonder why she had to straighten her hair at all, when it's so difficult to work with afterwards. It was so easy before to fix the hair with pins in tails that stayed nice and tidy all day.

Then I start realizing that wearing the rollers isn't for the end result, but that in Victoria's opinion it's fine as it is. A head surrounded by curlers is the most beautiful sight there is. For the first time in her life Victoria has curlers in her hair. She has been watching jealously how women curl their hair around big pink curlers. Now she can do the same herself.

It's just like my childhood, when I was dreaming of the time when I could wear high-heeled shoes. How fine it felt to drag my feet along in mother's too big, but wonderfully high-heeled shoes.

Yes, I understand Victoria, but I get so tired of looking at her round pink astronaut helmet day after day!

One afternoon I'm taking a rest while Anderson works in the garden and Victoria is in the kitchen. Joppe has gone to the hotel swimming pool. A car drives into the yard; it's Dr. King's wife, one of the active women at the Yacht Club. I go get pen and paper, and the lady writes her business.

Joppe should leave for the Sailing Competition with the Yacht Club Team flying to St. Vincent. The plane leaves in an hour from the airport.

In an hour! It's impossible! But this certainly is something Joppe has been looking forward to—it will be his big opportunity! I tell Mrs. King we'll try our best. Anderson runs to the pool to get Joppe. Victoria collects Joppe's clothes, helping me, and we pack them into a bag. But I don't have any money, and Joppe's passport is in the Barclay Bank's safe. We have to call up Jukka. Victoria dials the number. Jukka is not in the office, but Victoria leaves a message that he should contact home immediately.

In fifteen minutes Jukka drives with whistling wheels into the yard, looking pale. Then he's furious when he realizes nothing serious was happening: Joppe and I are fine. Jukka gives Victoria a strong lecture: don't leave those kinds of telephone messages. You must say what it's all about.

Victoria listens seriously, but after Jukka has left with Joppe to get the passport and then go to the airport, Victoria bursts out laughing. She pantomimes how fast Jukka was driving when he swerved into the yard.

"Your husband gets angry easily!" she repeats. Yes, Jukka has a hot temper and gets angry easily, even though he looks so gentle.

"You understand, don't you, that he loves me. Even if I don't always wear shoes inside!" And Victoria laughs again, but Anderson nods seriously.

Now, however, Joppe is sailing at St. Vincent. After a few days he returns, carrying a small goblet with him, and it will certainly be his most beloved souvenir from St. Lucia. Joppe also wins a plate in the series competition at the St. Lucia Yacht Club, but he doesn't tell us very much about his sailing.

Zenia visits to show us her baby. She stands on the road between the flamboyant and the oleander with a baby in one arm, holding a big black umbrella. I take Jeri inside and wave for Zenia to come in. She sits on the balcony, pale with black shadows under her eyes, happy and shy, the baby prettily dressed in pure white clothes. Zenia is one of those motherly types to whom giving birth and caring for children is easy and natural. She doesn't worry too much about the future. Today one of the fathers has given her money for food; tomorrow is tomorrow.

The baby is a boy, thin-faced and very light-skinned. No wonder Anderson doesn't quite accept the baby as his own! But Jukka demands that Anderson give Zenia money whether the child is his or not.

Jeri is barking continuously in the bedroom, and I tell Zenia that Jeri has to come and greet them, otherwise he won't stop barking and will become angry. He'll dash out of the bedroom looking wild, but she shouldn't worry about that. He'll sniff her for a while, and then go to sleep on the living room floor.

Jeri dashes out barking and starts sniffing Zenia and the baby. Zenia goes pale and draws the baby closer; that beast will eat her baby, for sure! But Jeri soon loses interest and goes into the living room to lie down.

Victoria bustles about with soup and tea for Zenia. "You have to drink tea so you'll have enough milk for the baby."

Zenia eats; the soup is really delicious, Victoria knows that.

"I don't know how to cook," Zenia says longingly.

She knows already that she won't get her job back. Victoria cooks well and isn't even afraid of the dog.

"If you need help, you ask for me; tell Anderson." I push a bag of food into Zenia's hand. "You can come some day to wash clothes. Victoria cooks, and you wash the clothes."

I have to help Zenia, who has five mouths to feed, a baby in her arms, and black shadows under her eyes—it hasn't been easy for her.

But when Zenia has left, Victoria says, "Madame, my sister knows how to wash clothes. She could come here!"

Doesn't Victoria realize that I don't need a washing woman now, but that I want to help Zenia? Now she is pushing her sister forward to wash for me! I don't understand Victoria's way of thinking.

BACK TO SCHOOL

One day Alfonso comes home with a hole in his lip—it looks as if a tooth has pierced it. The wound is bleeding and there's blood on his shirt. He stands in front of me looking proud and defiant, but crying at the same time. Alfonso says that Clyde threw him onto the ground, and his lip was pierced by a tooth. I guess that the boys have been quarreling, and Clyde has tried to restore order.

I've been thinking of starting to teach at the school again. It doesn't seem to do me any good just to stay home.

One afternoon I ride with Jukka when he drives to town after lunch. The door to the classroom is open, but nobody notices the car stopping in front of the building. Everybody seems to be deep in hard work.

When I step into the classroom, the girls see me and clap their hands happily. It feels so good that I cheer up at once. Even the boys are looking up from their work.

The girls have a lot to tell me. They sign and explain, and gradually the boys join in. Clyde also comes to greet me and explains that there's a new girl in the class, Magilda.

Magilda is a big sturdy girl, about 15 years old, who looks quiet and calm. She looks at me appraisingly, because she doesn't know me yet.

"I was angry at you some time ago," I tell Clyde. I have to clear up the matter at once.

"Why?" Clyde looks surprised, but he knows what it's all about.

"Roger came home from school one day with his lip split and said that you had thrown him on the ground. In my opinion the teacher should never do that."

Of course Clyde has his own view on the subject. And so do all the others.

The incident seems to have overturned the whole school, because as the day goes by I get to hear many different versions of it. When I am left alone in the classroom with a woman from the Red Cross, she starts explaining events. I get the story from her gestures, although I don't understand anything of her speech. When I go outside, the smaller children are around me at once, telling me the story.

But I don't know and never will know the exact truth of the matter.

Kenneth had provoked Alfonso, maybe pulled the chair out from under him when he intended to sit down. That kind of situation is quite humiliating to the victim, who finds himself sitting on the floor. Alfonso got mad, and the boys started to quarrel. Clyde told them to go outside. Kenneth is used to being thrown out or threatened with being sent home, but not Alfonso. He doesn't agree to leave, especially when he hasn't done anything wrong. Kenneth started it all. Clyde tries to push him outside, but Alfonso fights back, and a scuffle begins, during which Alfonso falls on the floor, and his tooth pierces his lip.

After this, Alfonso goes out and stands defiantly on the grass in front of the school. It starts raining, harder and harder, but Alfonso just stands there until he is soaking wet. I can imagine him standing there with his head up, full of spite, with every muscle hardened, his gaze walled in by rage, lip bleeding, and finally the whole boy dripping wet.

Alfonso's impossible pride is, in the end, at the bottom of everything. What a long way it is from this defiant and arrogant Alfonso to that smiling Alfonso whom I have made contact with a few times by pure chance!

How wonderful he must have felt over my comforting! But on the other hand, no power in the world could have persuaded Alfonso to change his opinion: Clyde bad. School bad.

Later, when Alfonso's defiance vanishes, it seems as if he has forgotten it all, as if nothing had happened.

Clyde has to give up his ambitious curriculum. The children haven't been able to adapt to it, which is understandable. Of course they get tired of copying a text in which they understand only a few words, one grasping more, the others less; a text with so many new words in it. But how can they be taught science and religion with the methods used in a regular school? How can we help them understand the world around them? Clyde builds equipment for making observations. I laugh when I see how full he has filled the classroom while I've been away!

It seems that the children only have enough interest and energy for one or two hours of work. In the beginning of the term they had more energy, but now they start getting tired after an hour or two—there's no way to prevent it. They're restless, glancing more and more often at what's happening outside. Victor plays and laughs and attracts the others' attention more and more; Clyde's hand bangs the table harder and more often . . . No, now it's time to do something else—draw, paint, sew, do crafts.

Clyde tells me his troubles, and I tell him that he shouldn't feel bad at all. It's not his fault that the children don't have enough language to acquire new knowledge, that they have come to school so late, and are in school only a couple of hours each day. They should have been signed to since they were small. This phase, when they have only a few dozen learned concepts should have been over ten years ago. Every concept would add to their possibilities for expanding their vocabulary, and at the same time their range of knowledge. It would be like numbers being squared, a geometric increase. But the children are like a heavy engine at the station, only barely getting started. You can't expect the locomotive to start moving a hundred miles an hour right away.

effects of lack of education

We think that now when the children are in school for their last year, they should learn all the things they'll need most for their everyday life. But what kind of information and skills will they need? What will their lives be like?

In this community with its open doors, where everything happens outside, the deaf person is usually included in everything. He sees before his eyes the whole of life, he dances on the streets with others during carnivals and other celebrations, feels the solemn devout spirit of the Catholic churches. But does he take in all these wonders with round eyes like Theresa, or get frustrated like Kenneth? The life of a deaf person over here includes lots of taking part, which gives better possibilities for communication than in countries where people are more reserved, but here deafness also means being isolated because deafness is not yet understood on the island.

same & diff as in other countries

We agree that I will teach the girls handiwork and home economics, shopping, how to use money, the names of food ingredients, the most important facts about nutrition; these skills are really needed. I could take the girls home to cook. There are only four of them, so it would work fine. At the same time the girls would learn setting the table, sewing, and table manners. What for? Well, they might be able to work in a restaurant or a hotel.

I am anything but a household and handicraft person, but I teach the girls all I know and find books for the rest. We don't get very far, however. A year ago, the girls couldn't even hold a needle in their hands, and doing handiwork was difficult in every respect, as if they weren't mature enough for it. But now they've changed a lot, and I can try again. This had all been in the curriculum even before I left, but at that time the day always ended before we ever got to handiwork or home economics.

After school I go to town and buy yarn and crochet hooks, fabric and sewing needles.

I return home filled with enthusiasm and eagerness. How on earth have I been away from school even a day? It's so awfully interesting there that sometimes it's hard to keep my wits about me.

This is the feeling I always have back home when I return from an event for the deaf, where there were no barriers to communication or to one's self-expression. How wonderful it felt! There were none of the hindrances that the hearing world is so full of, that make one creep down inside one's skin smaller than before, instead of bursting out of it! ❧

why does she feel good in this sit?. She has trouble w/ communicating w/ them!

"TELL THAT BOY"

Sunday afternoons I give Alfonso a dollar to go to the movies. But now he goes to an earlier show and comes home while we're still sitting on the balcony drinking tea after dinner. He doesn't come home and knock on the door at midnight any more. Jukka laid down the law so effectively that for once it was clear! Jukka thinks that Alfonso understands more than I suspect, and when he does something wrong he does it consciously. He understands what he's told. I don't know, could be. I've never seen intentionality behind my own boys' tricks, although Jukka has. Jukka has more common sense than I do; my overwhelming motherly instinct sometimes makes me blind!

Alfonso is usually enthusiastic about what he has seen; he tells me all about the movie. I'm always surprised at the new expressions he uses while telling each story. At school Clyde has talked about plants, and now Alfonso tells me about a big plant that has stretched its leaves and swallowed an entire person. The movie was horrible, as usual. Alfonso shows how throats had been cut, stomachs split, people hanged. Alfonso's gestures and facial expressions are effective. When he shows how the rope has been put around the throat, he looks just like a person being hanged.

What kind of trash do they show over here? I doubt very much that these films are at all suitable for Alfonso, Kenneth, and Victor. Besides, they only see it, they don't know anything that's being said.

After watching these movies for many Sundays, Alfonso starts telling me about his nightmares. He is afraid to go to his room and to bed. Somebody could creep into his room and put a rope around his neck. He is quite sure that somebody is sneaking around outside his room at night. The light from the street lamp that reflects from the road shows a pair of feet sneaking behind the door. Alfonso can see them from under his door, and he's afraid.

He tells this in the afternoons to Victoria and me. He seems to be combining the horror stories from the movies with the ones from his life—a mixture of dream, reality, and the myths and superstitions of the island.

It became clear to me that Victoria understands Alfonso's gestures better than I do, maybe because she has always lived on the island and knows its life. But she also finds a solution to what Alfonso's "tomorrow-tomorrow-tomorrow" means. In his language, it doesn't mean the future, but the past. I wonder if tomorrow-tomorrow for Alfonso is any time that isn't just now?

I react to Alfonso's fears as seriously as I did to Joppe's and Keke's fears when they were small. "Let the light stay on," Keke said when he was small, and I let the light shine all night long.

But I can't help in any concrete way. I don't know if somebody really has been sneaking around outside Alfonso's door. It is possible, but probably it's just been the neighbor's cat or dog wandering around. Alfonso is getting dream and reality mixed up, or is imagining. It's easy to see something fearful in the shadows of trees and bushes and light poles, especially when he has just seen a movie whose primary intention is to inspire horror in the people who watch it.

I assure Alfonso that Jeri doesn't let anybody come near the house. He barks, and then the Man-Who-Carries-Briefcase takes a flashlight and goes to look. Alfonso locks the door; nobody gets in to cut his throat or to put a rope around his neck.

I can only make the decision that Alfonso cease going to the movies, at least not every Sunday. When I tell this to Alfonso, he adjusts to it—to my great surprise—as if he's actually pleased.

Idleness is not good for Alfonso either. All our neighbors and friends assure us that we have to put him to work.

The worst flabbiness has really disappeared from the boy, but he still spends too much of his time just sitting on the balcony looking around.

Jukka sets Alfonso to taking care of the garden and washing the car. I tell him that he doesn't need to come to the balcony to wait for mealtimes, he'll get his meals on time.

To my joy Alfonso learns quickly to wash and wax the car, and he does it well, not like the boys at the garage where one boy is swishing the cloth carelessly, and the other one pours water from a bucket, often on a spot that the first boy has just dried. If nothing else, Alfonso knows now how to wash and wax a car and can earn something with that skill.

In gardening Alfonso is much cleverer than Anderson. We sow parsley and radishes, and Jukka is horrified when Alfonso goes and gets a bucket of cow dung and spreads it on the garden.

"Make sure that the boy washes his hands and the bucket as well. He did the right thing; cow dung is a good fertilizer, but do make sure that he washes his hands properly."

"Make sure that the boy does this and that; tell the boy this and that"!

I have told him and made sure! I've run after him, watched, and explained. It has been hard, and I haven't had enough energy to give Alfonso as much time as I should have. I know if I had had the strength to discuss everything with him, to teach and guide him, he would have learned much more.

Alfonso does have the will to converse and tell me about his thoughts and ask me things, because as soon as he notices that I'm alone, he comes and talks to me. When I'm with Joppe and Jukka, he knows that I can't focus my attention only on him.

I know my limitations as Alfonso's teacher, but my inner resources will allow me to do only so much. I'm groping in the dark. If I had some test, some method by which I could test Alfonso's nature and thoughts, it would be easier. And often I wonder whether I'm really helping Alfonso or whether it's the other way around.

Nowadays, though, it's much easier than it was in the beginning. Alfonso is at school; he'll learn more from his peers than from me. If I say something, he doesn't necessarily believe me, but when someone at school says the same thing, then he'll accept it. Also, Jukka is taking greater responsibility for the boy. It's not just "tell that boy" now, Jukka tells him himself. As they washed the car, Jukka and Alfonso developed some kind of contact, but I don't know what Alfonso thinks of Jukka's stern, absolutely commanding style.

Alfonso is inventive. He moves an okra plant from a rocky place into a smoother, shady place, where it soon starts to flourish. Again I am proud of the energetic Alfonso. When he comes home from school, he goes swimming. He runs and exercises on the beach and looks with satisfaction at his bulging muscles. For many months now, his stomach has been full of nourishing food. When he gets back from the shore, he washes the car or works in the garden. In the evenings he putters around in his room, cutting out pictures and learning to write. I stop in once in a while to watch and to guide. Maybe his hanging out on the balcony really was waiting for food. It's much nicer to be busy with something.

During the dark, rainy evenings as we sit on the balcony, thoughts ripen in my mind as if I'm reaching conclusions from my experiences. Nothing can ever completely open up the hearing world for me, that I now know. For that to happen, people would have to start conversing in writing, using an overhead projector or other visual means. Or everyone would learn sign language and would converse in sign language. This prerequisite can never be fulfilled, and even if it were, hearing people would still remain hearing, and deaf people, deaf. The world without sound is different. Nobody can do anything about that.

Parties will always be energy-draining and more or less frustrating, tedious occasions. But I'm learning to change my attitude. I don't feel like flinging the glass from my hand and fleeing any more. I know now how to handle the "glass in the hand" situations that are the most frustrating.

Sometimes I sit for hours with people, either at home or somewhere else. It's easy at home; most of the time goes for serving. Sometimes Jukka interprets something and I answer, sometimes I try to think of something to say. During these hours I don't get any closer to the people who are visiting us; I don't get any kind of contact with them. When they leave, I look at them like dreamlike creatures, especially because during the last hour I've dwelt completely inside my own thoughts. Jukka usually doesn't have anything to interpret from these visits. Maybe I'm the same kind of formless creature to them as well.

Slowly I have learned to observe people when they speak and to draw my own conclusions. When I don't put all my energy into trying to snatch up words from their lips, I can see quite a lot from the way they talk, gesture, hold their hands. I have learned to distinguish the hostess style and guest style. I also notice hidden yawns (ah ha, not everybody is having a good time! Some would like to go home already!), looking at watches, quiet smiles, glances exchanged.

But I have only recently learned this. I haven't yet developed my observation of much beyond speech movements. I am completely empty when I come home, but in a different way than before. Then I had used up my whole battery-charge, and that's why I felt totally exhausted. Now I feel more naturally empty. The greater part of my energy is still there, but I haven't gained anything new, no new thought or opinion. It's just as if we hadn't been anywhere at all. The whole story can be closed like a door behind you without a memory of where you came from. It's a strange feeling, like a dream. There's only one relief left, when after tight, high-heeled shoes you can change into sandals and sink, relaxed, onto the couch.

All the people in this dream world are not formless in the same way: some carry the potential for human contact. Sometimes I meet a person with whom I feel I make contact right away. And there are also people with whom I know I could form a contact if we had a way to share our thoughts.

These party people from the dream world are somehow unique. They are like different people every time we meet; there's no continuity. Well, in a way they become more familiar, gradually, slowly, when Jukka finally tells me later what these people have said. Often I realize that there was no point in being anxious, and I feel sorry that I didn't know what they said. The people in the dream world had halos, before; they stood on pedestals, higher than me, and when they said something, I thought they were saying something that was noble and worthy of respect.

It was I who thought I lacked a halo; I sat beneath the pedestals looking up to those others without saying anything. But little by little I have learned that halos and pedestals are all illusion—that we are all the same kind of people, in the end. 🌐

PEPSI, NO

Finally the heat of the sun lets go and we feel the cooling breath of the longed-for northeastern trade winds. Then the heavy-rain period begins in November. It doesn't rain nearly as much as it did the year before, but still the rain limits our comings and goings, and absences from school increase.

We're sitting beside the table in the classroom, the girls with crochet hooks in their hands. Finally I've been able to teach them something—they know how to crochet! Filipa has crocheted baby slippers, because the girls are so endlessly interested in babies and their clothes. The whole class is proud of the baby slippers Filipa has produced.

While we crochet, water starts dripping through the ceiling. The rain outside pours down harder and harder. We move to another place in the room until the drops from the ceiling drive us away, and soon they aren't drops any more, but streams of water; the whole roof is leaking like a sieve. We get buckets and cans for the worst places, move notebooks, papers, and pictures to a safer spot. Even the leaky roof is still a kind of shelter now that heaven is emptying all its reservoirs and water is forcing itself in everywhere. People take cover under shelters; the deserted park has turned into a lake that sends rushing cascades down onto lower areas.

We stand at the door; the sight of the rain draws like a magnet. Nobody says anything, everyone just watches quietly. We watch the rain slow down and gradually end.

During the downpour the neighboring schools have closed, and we must start cleaning up the classroom. We see the boys in uniforms from the neighboring school trying to wade through the lake, but it's impossible. The boys turn back after one of them loses his shoe, buried in the mud.

Fortunately I've asked Jukka to give me a ride home. I have to wait a long time for him. In the meantime the water level in the park has fallen; the grass is still muddy, but cars are driving on the asphalt roads.

What a traffic chaos! The traffic is completely confused; the streets in town are all flooded. Although the street-side ditches are deep, the drains can't take in water as fast as they should during the downpours. For half an hour we can't get out of the park. But then an inventive pedestrian starts directing traffic, and he gives the right-of-way in turn to those of us coming from the park.

Joseph and Alfonso are sitting patiently in the back seat. Joseph often comes to visit us after school. I'm happy that Alfonso has a friend. From Victor, Alfonso learns exaggerated signs that, just because they're exaggerated, make Alfonso sure that these are the ones he should use. From Kenneth, Alfonso learns aggressive behavior and squabbling; from Joseph, to balance it all, calm behavior. Alfonso's peers affect him much more than I do, and if I've influenced his life a bit, I've at least seen to it that Alfonso doesn't need to be alone any more; now he has friends.

I buy fabric for the girls to use to sew aprons and scarves.

I tell them that soon we'll go to my home to cook.

"All?" The girls' hands draw a wide circle.

"No, the boys stay here, only the girls cook."

The girls look satisfied. They know how to do something that the boys can't be a part of!

The girl's hand jumps up now from the cheek outwards, the thumb leading.

"Tomorrow?"

No, not tomorrow. I take the girls to the calendar and show them the date.

The girls' fingers are making walking movements, first through the park, then up the opposite hill.

"No, we won't walk, we ride in a car." My hands turn an imaginary steering wheel.

"Red?"

The girls have seen a red Mini bringing me to school and coming to pick me up.

The girls are already all excited, but first we learn theory. I put macaroni, flour, sugar, coffee, and other dry ingredients into small jars. We examine them and learn their names.

I tell them how important cleanliness is in the kitchen. One has to have clean hands and fingernails, and clean dishes. There can't be festering cuts on the hands; when one is coughing or has a stuffy nose one should not cook. We go to the basin and wash our hands well. I remove chipped nail polish from Theresa's nails and give the girls nail brushes, manicure sticks, and clippers to use to clean and cut their fingernails. I tell them that they can't come to cook at our house with nails that are dirty or long. The hair has to be clean and the dress tidy.

Yes, yes. The girls show me how they fetch water and wash their hair. Valerie shows that she has shampoo in a bottle that she pours on her hair. We take care of all the small cuts on the girls' hands. I examine the girls' fingernails and handkerchiefs every day.

I write on the board, and the girls copy what I write. I know that copying is very mechanical, the girls won't learn anything from it, but we paste pictures in the notebook as much as possible, and when each girl has her colorful home economics notebook done, maybe she'll benefit from it, remember something from it—at least that the hands have to be clean when handling food ingredients.

My teaching of cleanliness seems to reach its goal, but when I try to teach the right kinds of nutrition, there's a wall facing me.

I explain what a bad lunch it is to have a bottled soft drink and a roll or a piece of cake. One doesn't get energy from them for work, and sweets are bad for the teeth. It would be better to drink water, to buy eggs, cheese, and fruit instead of soft drinks.

I show on the board how these two different lunches cost the same, but that the second one is much healthier.

"Pepsi, no?" Theresa is wondering. Never soft drinks?

The girls understand from my teaching only that they are not allowed to drink soft drinks. Everybody drinks Pepsi and red soft drink!

I leave the matter. I know that the diet of the islanders is not bad at all—a lot of fish and vegetables, little butter. But probably this diet doesn't have enough iron, calcium, or B vitamins in it, and lunch at work and school for the islanders often is only a bottle of soft drink and a roll without anything on it.

I write notes for the girls to take home: "The girls in the class will come to my house to cook on Wednesday. Please send some vegetables and fruit, whatever is growing in your yard, with your daughter."

On Tuesday the whole class goes grocery shopping at the J. Q. Charles and M. K. C. stores. We choose items, examine prices. Everywhere a crowd watches us.

The girls' families must not grow many vegetables or fruits, because when the girls get out of Jukka's car on Wednesday with their brown paper bags, they only have a few breadfruit, passion fruit, and coconuts with them.

The girls are shy. It's as if we were meeting for the first time. I put the bags in the kitchen and take the girls to wash their hands. I tie their new aprons around their waists and scarves over their heads. Victoria stops at the kitchen door and laughs. I introduce the girls: Valerie, Filipa, Theresa, and Magilda. This is Victoria, the woman who helps me, washes my dishes, cooks my food, and cleans up.

Victoria giggles. But she's a tremendous help when we start cooking. The girls peel, cut, grate, mash, mix. Everyone would like to do everything. Filipa is talented, skillful, and quick. Theresa is timid as always about doing anything without a thorough explanation. Magilda has just enough self-confidence, she is bright and a fast learner; she learned the finger alphabet in a couple of months and signs enough to talk to the others. Her reservedness has broken up a bit, she accepts me—but she doesn't accept very much guidance.

I show them the meanings of "to boil," "to fry," "to grill," and "to bake." I show how to measure ingredients. Ounces, pounds, pints, cups. I have to change all the recipes into those measures I know. St. Lucia is changing to the metric system gradually.

By noon we've prepared a vegetable salad, hamburgers, and different kinds of breadfruit dishes: fried, mashed, as a casserole; passion fruit juice to drink. For dessert, coconut pie.

The girls set the table and eat. I bring each of them the bottle of red soft drink that I promised them. I know this isn't the best diet, but I can't teach them everything at once.

The girls use a knife and fork clumsily. It's like a ceremony for them to eat at a table covered with a cloth, with napkins and flowers on it. Victoria eats in the kitchen behind the serving window and laughs. I don't understand why she laughs the whole time.

Sometimes Victoria brushes Alfonso's hair and looks carefully at his scalp as if to learn whether the fleas and worms have gone into his brains so that the boy, besides being deaf, is also dumb and completely stupid. Is that what she also thinks of me behind all her sweet talk?

The girls take a shower, comb their hair fussily, load themselves into the car for the drive back to school. I can see that they've had a fun day. I don't know if they've learned anything about cooking, but they've certainly experienced something new. They'll remember this "different" day.

I send a bottle of juice and a piece of cake to the boys. Clyde lets me know that the boys will always come and have lunch at my house on the girls' cooking days!

I sink into a chair. Whew!

"A very busy day," giggles Victoria.

"Yes, it was, but a nice one. Didn't you enjoy teaching home economics?"

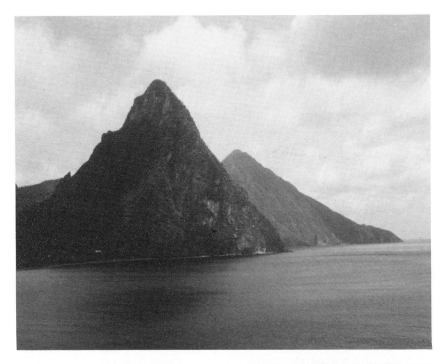

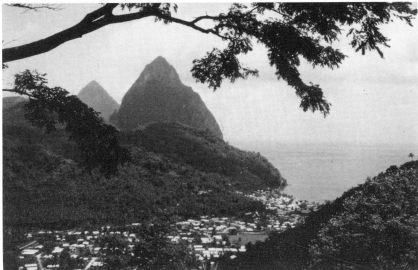

The Gros and Petit Piton volcanic islands can be seen clearly from St. Lucia.

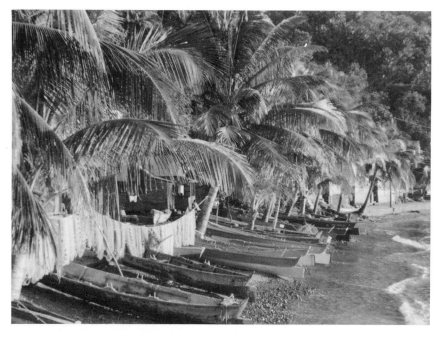

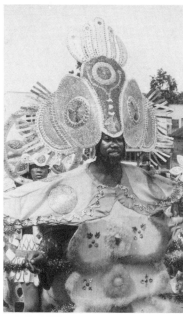

Our first few months were spent taking in the sights of the island. Above: the fishing boats stored beneath the coconut palms in the town of Sou-friere. Left: The King of the Carnival Bands, part of the annual February Carnival.

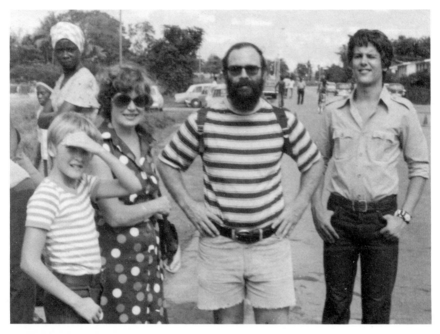

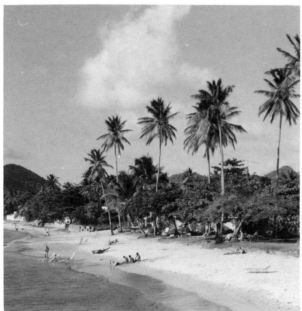

Left to right: Joppe, Raija, Clyde Vincent, and Keke on National Day, December 13, 1975.

The beach near Halcyon Beach Hotel where our family relaxed almost every afternoon after the workday.

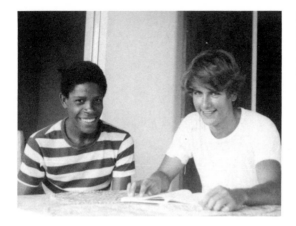

Keke (right) and his class-mate John Eugene (left) became great friends. John Eugene came over nearly every afternoon after school.

Clyde Vincent and his "babies" class in 1975.

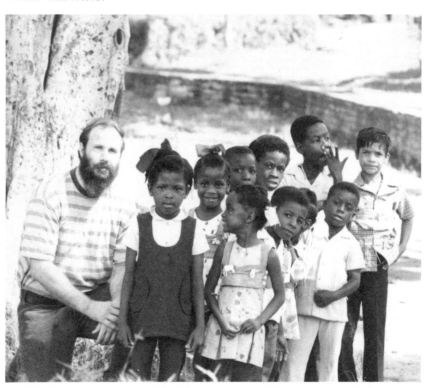

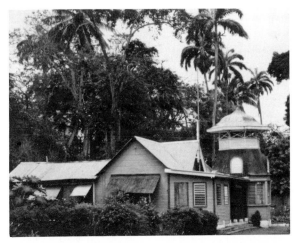

The ramshackle, but cozy, Red Cross building where the senior class studied during the 1976–1977 school year.

The senior class of 1977. Bottom row, left to right: Filipa, Valerie; middle row, left to right: Theresa, Kenneth, Victor; top row, left to right: Gregory, Alfonso, Joseph.

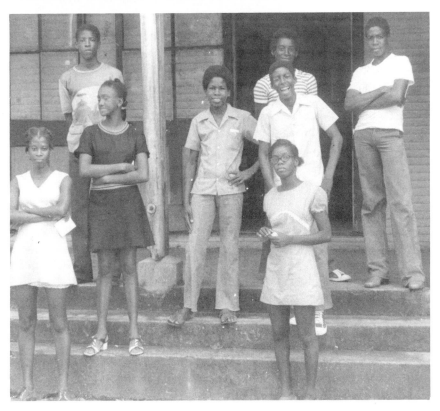

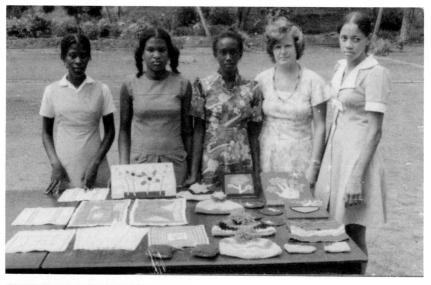

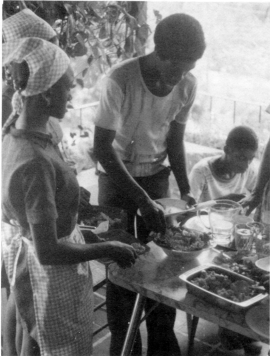

Above: Filipa, Magilda, and Theresa (left to right) display the handicrafts they made in school, with Roselyn's (far right) and my help.

Left: The senior girls learned to cook in my kitchen, and the senior boys offered to eat everything they made.

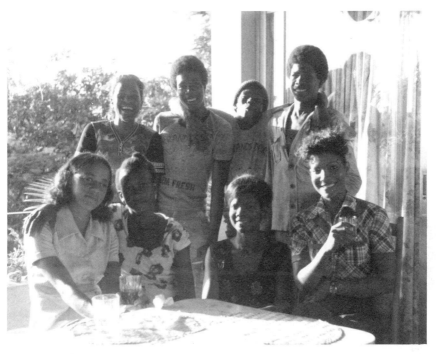

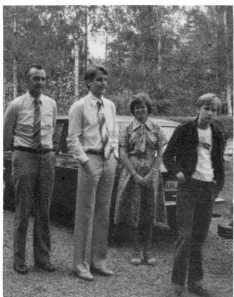

After the seniors graduated, they all found jobs. Every Wednesday they came to visit me and we formed "the Wednesday club." Seated left to right: Roselyn, Theresa, Arlette, Kathleen; standing left to right: Magilda, Joseph, Victor, Kenneth.

The family in Finland after Keke's high school graduation in 1979.

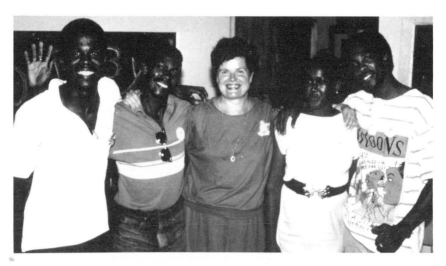

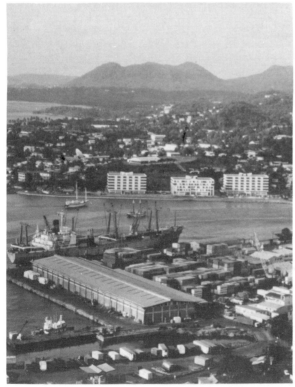

Jukka and I returned to St. Lucia in 1989. The St. Lucia School for the Deaf had a party for me, where I was able to see many of my former students; left to right are Kenneth, Victor, me, Theresa, and Joseph.

Left: The port of Castries in 1989. The warehouse, container yard, and two deep berths were built between 1975 and 1979, when Jukka was General Manager of the Port Authority.

CHRISTMAS ON
ST. LUCIA AGAIN

I have only a month and a half at school before Christmas vacation starts. Joppe gets good grades. The headmaster said that Joppe could move up one grade after Christmas, because his English is going so well. It won't take long for him to be up to the same grade he'd be in back home. But Joppe will leave now to go to school in Finland.

I read Joppe's essays and wondered where he learned all those words. He writes that "we" should do this or that to improve the St. Lucia economy, and I notice that besides being skilled in picking out words and phrases from speech, he has also listened carefully when Jukka has discussed his work in the evenings! Joppe has been listening with burning eyes. Maybe he will one day be as strong, exact, and demanding as Jukka is. At least he shows that in his relationship with Alfonso: a matter-of-factness, never much emotion. From Victoria he knows how to demand service better than I can.

"Since we have a maid, she can fix me some juice."

Joppe is loosening the ties to mother, politely but firmly. And maybe later on he, too, will need a quiet and gentle wife who has time and energy to listen to his work worries in the evenings.

We're having a Christmas party at school. The children are all excited. Some parents and relatives have also arrived. There's a Santa Claus picture drawn on the board. Under the Christmas tree there's a gift for every child and food is ready on trays in the back room.

Clyde leads games; the children are noisy, they eat cakes, ice cream, sandwiches—they're enjoying themselves. How different this Christmas party is from those I had in my childhood on dark winter mornings when Christmas carols echoed in the big classroom of the wooden schoolhouse and made chills run up my spine. It was so devout, and festive, and Christmas-like. Over here the atmosphere is never devout or festive. Christmas-like it can be, but for people over here the Christmas atmosphere is different. There is so much going on, so much dance and music.

But for the children the packages under the tree are the most important thing. It's important that there is a package for everyone with the right name written on it. Rattling of paper and yelling, dolls, cars, balls. The presents are taken to the relatives who sit in the back, and then the children go and continue their games. Everybody watches Alfonso bring his ball to me . . . I am the mother, the woman who cares.

To understand a deaf child demands knowledge, help, guidance.

The pupils often show off Victor's chin: on it is "a map of the neighbor island," a big burn-scar that resembles the big island.

His mother got angry and burned his chin with a cigarette.

It's quite possible, although you can't always believe what the children are telling you.

Kenneth is telling us constantly that his current "mother" is bad, hits him, does not give him food. Kenneth is always begging for money and food, and I won't give it to him because I don't completely believe him.

But it is very probable that one of the mothers has become very angry when she's been unable to make her poor, speechless child understand even the simplest thing. She has completely missed getting any information about the child's potential.

Now the situation is better than before, when Victor and Kenneth were small. Now the parents can come to the school with their deaf child. Hearing will be tested, parents guided—they aren't alone any more. They get support.

The next day we go to the beach for a "beach party." The weather is rainy; once in a while there's a cool rain shower, and the wind blows. I'm cold; I hold little Albert, one of the younger children, on my lap.

I walk along the shore near the house. There are sad-looking dogs running on the sand, thin and full of fleas. They wag their tails and beg for food and friendliness, but I don't want to touch them, no matter how much I like dogs or how sorry I feel for them.

I pass the small zoo. I've heard that in the zoo a snake and a mongoose fight, but I've never seen visitors there. The owner is ambitious. On the shore by the zoo there's a small cafe where food and drinks are being served. "Hygienic," the sign assures us. Every time I pass the cafe something new has appeared there. Now there's a big barrel of rum punch and halves of barrels as chairs and tables; necklaces made of shells are hanging on dead tree branches. Girls are selling similar necklaces on the beach.

Beside the zoo the fishermen have beached their colorful boats. They have just recently returned from the sea and are lifting a beautiful, rainbow-colored lobster from the boat.

"How much?"

Four fingers rise: four dollars.

Only four dollars, yet a portion of lobster costs tens of dollars in the restaurant.

"Good?" I ask Alfonso—he knows these sea creatures.

Alfonso is nodding eagerly; I can see that his mouth is almost watering.

I pay four dollars to the fisherman, and Alfonso grabs the creature skillfully, away from the stickers, or are they scissors?

What a beautiful animal.

Alfonso is carrying the lobster proudly past the hotel. The tourists on the beach are looking at him with surprise.

A big surprise is that there are tourists in the hotel; mostly it's been empty and deserted. I wonder if better times are dawning for tourism on the island? Hopefully the island won't be spoiled; it's one of the only unspoiled areas in the whole world.

"Do you know how to cook lobster?" I ask Victoria.

Of course Victoria knows how. She knows how to cook crabs, mollusks, and everything from the sea. Once she brought mollusks from the market and cooked them, but none of us ate them. For Alfonso she cooked a big plateful of snails spiced with salt and lemon. Thank you, but no thank you, not for us.

Victoria puts the beautiful, rainbow-colored lobster into a bucket and pours hot water over it. It flaps and splashes water until it turns red and stops flapping. Victoria lifts it into a pan and cooks it and doesn't mind a bit.

But whew! That's the last time I'll buy a lobster, no matter how good it is, even if it were the greatest delicacy in the world. If it's up to me, the creatures can stay where they belong. Let them stay alive and keep their beautiful color.

And besides, there's so little to eat in one lobster, as I see when Victoria puts the meat on a dish and decorates it with mayonnaise, tomatoes, lettuce, and eggs. There's not much for four people, and Alfonso is waiting for his portion with watering mouth!

The next day Victoria prepares a casserole from breadfruit and minced meat. I begin to wonder how Victoria has used up so many eggs! It was just yesterday that I bought thirty, I remember clearly, and now there are only thirteen left. How about the milk and butter? Out of the weekly portion over half is gone.

When Victoria comes to work on Monday, she has a baby with her! Did she suspect something when I counted eggs and searched through cupboards, wondering?

But the child won't soften me. I must know.

I can't manage Victoria; she will win me over again. Jukka is leading the discussion. Because food costs are so high, and prices are rising all the time, we want to know where so much milk and so many eggs are going. We need to start thinking how costs can be reduced.

I expect Victoria to explain: "Madame, don't you remember that eggs were needed to decorate the lobster, so many for the casserole, and so many for the meatloaf."

But she doesn't say anything like that at all. She tells an unbelievable story about how Alfonso came in while she was washing clothes, took the key from under the pillow on the balcony, and fried eggs and drank milk.

And then Victoria becomes hysterical. She shrieks and scolds, shouts and rages. I can only fling up my arms with surprise. Is this the same soft-spoken, religious, smiling person who has worked with us for months?

Nothing will be cleared up about the eggs, but if it's Victoria's habit to have these outbursts, we can't keep her. Jukka puts a check in Victoria's hand and drives her to town.

On the way Victoria calms down a bit and explains that she would have taken such good care of Jukka while Madame was back home. She even intended to send the children to the country for that time. Was her hair-straightening for that? What would all that "care" have included? I am amused and enraged, but in a way I feel free at the same time. It's as if I've been freed from something pressing me down. I really couldn't imagine what that girl kept inside her, how much rage and aggression. But somehow I was always so uncertain of her. Where have these people gotten their dual nature?

Anderson takes a message to Zenia that she can come to work for us, as before.

Zenia comes, and I feel wonderful when I smell the gas from the kitchen, a sign of Zenia having remembered to put the water on to boil. The kitchen and the whole house will be cleaned right on schedule. At noon the house is clean, clothes are hanging on the clothesline, drinking water is in the bottle, and Zenia is in the kitchen frying chicken for dinner!

I don't realize how close it is to Christmas already. Christmas decorations have appeared in the stores by now, but nothing else reminds us that Christmas is getting close. Christmas over here doesn't mean the same kind of awful hurry as back home. And besides, I'm going to Finland to take Joppe to school, and this supersedes all the Christmas preparations.

We'll have a guest for Christmas from Finland. This time it's my mother who comes to visit us. The boys mean everything to Granny—that's why she was so terrified when we said that we were leaving for the faraway Caribbean.

Now we show her that we don't live under primitive conditions. We show her the beauty of St. Lucia, its gorgeous beaches, rain forests, sunshine, flowers. We look at the sulphur springs where black water is bubbling, threatening—reminding us of the volcanic origin of the islands. We visit Diamond Falls and the old mineral baths that were founded by one of the French King Ludvigs.

I am leading my mother into the new world I've found over the past several years. I know that she's worried about the "matter of my hearing," but what could she have known or done earlier, back then—even though she might have suspected something—at a time when disabled people were not allowed to exist? Not until recently has it been understood that the parents of hearing-impaired children need a lot of support and help. Now my mother can see that everything is fine. The deaf world has opened up new possibilities for me.

Joppe is bustling with home-going gifts. For a year he has planned what he would take to his friends as presents, and now that the moment is here, he can't find anything. Joppe asks worriedly how much money he can spend on the gifts and runs around town searching for them. We collect shells and pieces of coral to take with us, and when Alfonso sees what we're doing, he concentrates all his energy on collecting shells. One day when we get back from town, the whole yard is full of shells sorted out in pretty piles, every species in its own. There are beautiful big shells among them like none we've ever found. But Alfonso knows the beaches and reefs and rock holes as only a few people do.

We look at the shells, admire them, and cry out with delight. Alfonso looks happy and satisfied. Joppe chooses the most beautiful shells and asks if he can pay for them. He digs dollars out of his pocket, but Alfonso shakes his head. No, Joppe can have them, he won't take any money.

I look at Alfonso, surprised. Has he finally learned what giving a present means? That there's actually something where money doesn't change hands, that there are even bigger concerns than receiving money? I don't know. Maybe Alfonso is in good spirits because he has just received new pants, completely new, not ones made smaller from somebody else's.

Alfonso happily and proudly took me into a shop that had his dream pants in its window. Maybe he's been secretly visiting to look at them through the window. They were expensive fashion jeans, and I couldn't buy them. Jeans were just making their way onto the island, so they were too expensive. But in the end Alfonso was as satisfied with the usual neat pants he got.

Yes, getting ready for Christmas is simpler here than back home. Zenia keeps the house tidy with her daily cleaning, which she does thoroughly. Anderson waxes the floors three times a year and washes the windows. Anderson has waxed floors in his other jobs, so he knows how to do it. I just have to make sure he takes off the dirt spots and the old wax first.

The rainy season has ended, and the humidity has dropped to 50 percent. The sun sets at the left of the lighthouse, and the evenings are lovely and fresh. I pack my suitcase and ponder that I don't have such a great urge to leave for Finland any more. It has happened like this many times before: I plan for the trip, but when departure time really is here, I don't want to leave.

Joppe is angry about the expression that I will "take" him home to our country. He is the one who goes—nobody needs to take him. Joppe is right. With his English skills he gets through changing planes much better than I do, so it's he who takes me from one plane to another. But what I meant by "taking" was that there is so much to be arranged back home. It's December, and Joppe doesn't have any winter clothes. Everything has to be bought from scratch. I have to see how the boys get on with their lives in the home country.

Now that we have friends over here, we get a lot of food as presents, according to the St. Lucia customs. Cornell brings two frozen turkeys, Maureen a sherry-flavored cake. The Daniels send the Christmas drink of St. Lucia, sorrel drink. Peter Paul kills a pig at his farm and brings us ham and sausage. Simon Richards, the boss at the port, brings a live rooster! It's a sign of friendship, and we're proud of it, but the rooster is crowing in the tool shed downstairs and I can't wring its neck and pluck it! Eugene takes care of it and brings the rooster, all plucked to Zenia.

We try to have a traditional Christmas like back home, but Christmas peace does not lie upon the island, not during the Christmas night nor the whole Christmas season.

We've been invited for two-thirty in the morning to a party at Merle Alexander's. She's our friend George's fiancée. But we just can't go out to a Christmas party in the middle of the night.

We have our Christmas dinner. Alfonso comes to the table all clean, with his curls greased. He reminds me of a Christmas angel. The neighbors go to church at midnight, and stay up all night after that eating, drinking, and dancing.

In the morning when we wake up, people are dancing on the balcony at the Barnards's house nearby. Soon people will leave for church wearing white clothes; after the mass there's a party again, and after this another one—for many days and nights. It's a matter of honor to stay awake.

On Christmas Day nausea puts me to bed, and it can't be eased at all. We have to call Dr. King to see if I can still take the trip. A situation where you don't know what to do is always the worst. Luckily our doctor is always friendly and helpful. After examining me he says that he can't recommend the trip. Okay, then. Jukka cancels my flight, and I submit with surprising ease to the fact that I can't leave. I've noticed many times how everything has its meaning.

I stay in bed and take medicine. Granny cooks. On the second day of Christmas, Joppe and Granny will leave. I'll travel when I'm in shape for it. My sister-in-law Leena promises to buy winter clothes for Joppe and take care of the boys. When I leave, my most important goal is to see Keke, whom I haven't seen for seven months.

"I had on a new shirt and a tie, my first tie, when I went to the airport; it was a surprise. And then Mother didn't come . . ." Keke writes.

Keke, standing behind the glass wall of the airport looking like a grown man, waiting for Mother's reactions!

When I'm over the worst of it, I go and open the door for Alfonso when he comes for breakfast.

"I saw no Raija. Man brought food."

"Me sick. Not go with Joppe. I go later."

Alfonso smiles and looks happy. Raija is still at home.

MYSTERIOUS VIRUSES

I want to know how much of all this that I experience will stay with me? Will I be a different person when I leave? Sometimes I feel as if information, experiences, and life experience have flowed into me until I'm completely full. Overwhelming impressions seem to stay in my mind. But sometimes I feel that there's nothing left, everything is gone, and the island is like any other place. I have become accustomed to everything, and I'm even fed up with much of it.

All that is so strange here, its very abundance, is exhausting. I have to withdraw and just exist for a few days, lying in a cool bedroom, reading. Why do I have to experience everything so intensely that sometimes I get absolutely, totally tired? Why can't I just float from one incident to another and be as lively the next moment as before?

When I actually fall ill, Jukka takes care that I don't keep jumping up. My viruses are usually mysterious. Dr. King examines my heart, lungs, throat, ears. Everything is fine, and yet I am sick, and those hidden viruses trouble me for a long time. Sometimes when the doctor presses my liver it's tender, and then the viruses have revealed their hiding place. The doctor prescribes medicine, but better are his sympathy and friendliness; he pats me, fatherly and encouraging: it will go away.

I lie there for days, looking at the blue sky outside, at the swaying palms and the red flowers glowing against the blue sky. In the afternoon I go and look through the balcony doors to the porch. It's quiet there; green lizards sleep or climb on the backs of chairs. The sea is shining. Later in the afternoon the sun is at such an angle that everything glows and shines—the sea, the palm fronds, all the green foliage.

It never rains when I'm sick. The bedroom could be anywhere when I'm a prisoner within its walls. I read and sleep, and sometimes I remember with surprise how close the port is, with its cruisers and colorful fishing boats. I think about the bay with sailboats swaying at anchor, the crowded marketplace, with its tumult and smells, the houses moping on stilts. The houses were built on the mountain slopes in the belief that there never would be earthquakes. I think about the noble tops of king palms at the top of the mountain.

I read, I think, I find things to do that will thrust me through the walls, over the garden, far, far. When I read, I see with new eyes these palms, the crabs crawling on the seashore, fruit trees bending, parrots shrieking in the rain forests. I write about everything like a person who sees all this for the first time, but the local writers write about things they have known since childhood. They see into the past and future; they see reasons and consequences.

I stare at brown water spots on the ceiling—new ones appear during the rainy season. Drops come down from the ceiling and the wind drives rain showers in through the window. I wake up often with the feeling that it's raining on my feet.

I look at the lizards that climb on the wrought-iron grid, catching insects. The house would feel deserted without them, charming pearl-eyed lizards snapping insects on the walls, dashing along the balcony rail or liana leaves, peering with their necks thrown backwards when I turn off the light.

At night after the lights have been turned out there are still bluish lights twinkling on the ceiling. The first time I got scared; it was as if the electric wire were sparking blue flames. I turned the lights on again and climbed on a chair to see. A firefly was crouching there, between the ceiling tiles. It didn't look like a fly at all, more like a beetle. After I turned off the light again it started descending toward me, sparkling along a spiral path. *Eeek.* I dived under my blanket.

Often my thoughts return to the past. All that is today depends on yesterday, and sometimes it's good to realize why something is as it is now. I am conscious that the borders of my life and views still are narrow, although lately they have broadened explosively. Maybe I started to grow too late—not until I entered the deaf world, and my communication possibilities grew.

I don't know what I would have become without Jukka. I met Jukka just when I was in an inextricable dilemma. The situation was completely critical. I needed help, but I didn't realize myself what kind of help I needed and what my problems were. I expected a miracle to happen. And it did.

Probably living on this island will also change me in many respects. The years to come will show how much.

Gradually my strength comes back. I want urgently to go to the beach, to feel the warm sand under my feet, to feel the heat of the sun pounding into my every cell, stimulating me. I want to drive to town and see people. And then when I go with Jukka in the evening, I experience again everything as new—the stooping fruit sellers along the streets in the dark, the rhythm of iron drums and beating feet, the smell of corn toasting on the coal pots, the lights from the open doors of the small rum stores, groups of men playing checkers and dominoes. This swarming life must produce a host of sounds; I only see the figures and shadows, I sense the smells and odors and quivering of drums. I can't hear the sounds, but I feel that there must be a lot of them.

It's as if I'm seeing everything for the first time again. Am I really on this island? How strange that life has thrown us here.

COLD DREAM

As evening draws near, I leave for the airport. Jukka can't come to see me off, but he has arranged a ride for me. The driver has instructions not to leave until he has seen me get onto the plane. Jukka has again sent letters and telexes; he's worried about my change of planes in London. Yes, it would be better to know that someone will help me do the changing. Heathrow is a difficult airport, and if one doesn't hear, one is quite insecure. I would be worried for the whole ten-hour flight to London.

But my mind is mellow as I look at the scenery of the island. The road winds through the valleys and mountains, the height differences are so great that my ears close up. Behind the valleys the sea is shining, those valleys with slopes on which the vegetation pours down almost like waterfalls. When you come to the shore of the Atlantic Ocean side, the scenery is rugged. On this side you can't swim, the shores are so steep and rough, full of reefs and jellyfish, or marshes and mud. The ocean is not turquoise like the west side, but cold, bright sapphire, spotted with bright white foam that strikes the sharp shore rocks and surges against the rugged bases of the cliffs.

The apple blossom cassias are starting to bloom and glow bright pink against the sky; it's just like midsummer at home with apple trees in bloom. The trees line the fields that the cows wander through. The trees were originally wire-fence poles, now grown into trees. Now the fences are bushy lines of trees; wires and rods are set crossways on their trunks.

Am I leaving this wonderful island? Do I have two homes, and don't know in which I want to live? Do I want to ski along shining spring snow and walk in the fall-fresh forest colored by autumn leaves, or walk along the yellow sand

culture
shock

under the swaying palms and blue sky, when brightly colored flowers are shining and the soft wind cools the heat of the sun?

We arrive at the airport early, the first ones at the check-in. We sit down to wait. The time passes comfortably. I have a cup of tea and watch people who are leaving as I am: tourists going back home, islanders to London. Relatives seeing people off, the travelers dressed in their best—and excited, handkerchiefs ready in their hands. Yes, leaving is not easy.

All of a sudden I feel sorry for those leaving. They will leave this beautiful, warm, home island where they get by the whole year in a light cotton dress, where they can pick mangoes from the trees, where air is unpolluted, and where people sit for hours in front of their houses, free of any hurry. They are going to the big city where it's cold and raw. They'll be cold there in the smoke, mist and rain, and unwarmed rooms, but above all, they'll be cold because they won't have their big family around them any more, dancing, laughing, warm, bursting: people who express their feelings.

Over there people don't smile on the streets as they pass you. There you must constantly look at your watch; it's all cold, hurry, and stress. I wonder if these people can stand stress, when they're so used to a peaceful life?

Oh, why do they leave? But the urge to leave is a powerful longing. Maybe they'll get used to all that's new over there in the new land. They'll get used to the city swarming with happenings, to the show windows, and the plentifulness of things, the flood of books, magazines, TV programs and information, movies— happenings, so many that time streams through your fingers. People are coming and going; you always have a feeling that there's so much to be done. Isn't it just this I've missed on the island, isn't it the reason I'm leaving now?

"Madame, the plane is landing right now. You have to go to the gate."

"Oh, thank you. Thank you for your help. I'll see you."

"Farewell. I won't leave before the plane leaves; I promised your husband."

Actually I didn't understand anything but the word "husband" from the last sentence, and from that I concluded what the whole sentence would be. It's just like my Latin exam at the University. I knew one word, guessed the rest, and translated the whole sentence. My life is one long Latin exam, full of guessing.

It's ten p.m. when the plane takes off. After half an hour it starts its landing

how she functions

— 215 —

on Antigua. Beneath us, light masses appear; the island must be flat and densely populated, because there are a lot of lights everywhere, and they don't climb up the hills. The mysterious island has sunk into the soft darkness except for its twinkling lights. The darkness hides everything that happens on the island. Maybe people are asleep there already.

There are so many more passengers getting on at Antigua that the plane is crammed full. A big fat man pushes himself in beside me. We take off, the lights of the island disappear, we're over the dark, cold Atlantic Ocean. There's a storm; the plane shakes and quakes.

What would I like to drink? The stewardness gestures. So she has been informed. A soft drink, please. But would I like wine with dinner? The steward-ess writes. Good girl, you are able to communicate; you get an A. Thank you, I'll have red wine.

People move their watches forward—something has been an-nounced. A-minus for this, good friends. Suppose there were a dangerous situa-tion and you announced it to the passengers, do you then leave me ignorant of the danger?

I look at my neighbor's watch. Four. And now a dinner is being served. I am not especially hungry. My stomach doesn't know if it's four o'clock or twelve o'clock, is it still in St. Lucia or already on London time?

I can't sleep. The man beside me takes up too much space; it's cold up here above the clouds; the plane shakes and jerks.

At nine o'clock breakfast is served. People line up for the toilet. I get cleaned up and pull some more clothes from my bag. We start to descend. I drag on a windbreaker and a poncho. I don't have winter clothes; I left them in Finland when we left.

The stewardess brings me a note that I should wait until I am escorted out. At the bottom of the stairs I stand and wait for my escort, shivering from cold next to two small boys. There's an icy, chilly wind in London.

We ride the bus to the front of the terminal. There's a nurse waiting for me! I don't remember afterwards whether there was also a wheelchair.

The nurse is embarrassed. I walk, I look normal, not like an invalid. Some-times it happens that my handicap is not understood at all. Oh, God, just take me to the right terminal and the right counter where I can show my ticket. But they don't seem to be able to understand such a simple matter. And I'm shivering from cold, carrying my bags under my poncho.

Blundering, blundering. I'm pushed from one person to another until I slip away and search out the plane for Finland myself. I won't accept these helping hands any more. Now that I've changed planes once in both directions, I already know how it works. And the second time I'll have my pen and paper ready. I am humiliated and angry, at myself as well because it was partly my own fault.

But this airport's personnel should be sent to a course for sure, to be informed what kind of help each disabled group needs, because I'm not the only one of the hundreds of thousands of people who use this airport and who need guidance.

In the domestic plane I order a brandy at once; it warms me up and lifts my spirits. Why on earth didn't I take my winter clothes along when I left Finland? It was November then, too! All the clothing that seemed so thick and warm on the island doesn't help much here in the cold. And this is only London—there isn't even any snow!

It feels wonderful to see my familiar mother tongue being spoken on the plane, to see familiar, fair-haired, blue-eyed people, to eat familiar food. I understand completely and easily every word the stewardess is saying. Have my lipreading struggles with English made it easier for me to lipread the language of my home country?

The plane lands on the dark, snowy, icy runway. I'm in the middle of the Finnish winter. I drag my poncho on and stumble in my thin shoes over the icy field to the terminal. Keke, Joppe, and Juha wait behind the glass wall—Keke in his new shirt and tie, with broader shoulders.

Keke hugs me heartily. I hardly reach to his shoulder any more. I remember when Keke was so small that when I said, "Show me how tall you are," he jumped on the bed to look taller. Joppe doesn't hug me. He looks annoyed when I hug him. Joppe thinks it's hardly necessary for him to come and greet me—it's just three weeks ago that we parted.

I quickly get used to the idea that it's winter now; I get used to the fact that the ground is covered with snow and the trees are leafless. But I'm constantly frozen. At night I dig myself under the quilt, I have a thick nightgown on, later I add socks and cardigan, shivering. My fingertips are stinging, my whole being feels shrunken. My body is used to warmth streaming from all around; now it can't get used to the sudden change of temperature.

It's also so cold mentally. People are in a hurry, their thoughts are on the money spent at Christmastime, on tax forms, and excess taxes in this period of depression. Their spirits are at the lowest ebb, now, after so many dark months, and it feels as if the sun has completely disappeared. At first it's hard for me to understand this gloomy atmosphere, because I still have the sunlight and warmth in my mind.

Kaisu visits me; she has a meeting at the Deaf Association, but I don't want to go along. "I'll come to see you, but don't wait for me," I write to Ella Mattila in Kotka. I don't go. When I even think of the bus ride through the dark, snowy scenery, I can't force myself to go. Gradually my mind sinks low. It's nice to be at home, in our cozy house with the relatives and the boys, but it's distressing even to think of going out the door. "Mother just sits at home, doesn't go anywhere," Keke writes to Jukka.

I do go get a new permanent and visit the Deaf Association office in Liisankatu. The office is moving to Olari to bigger quarters; there are boxes and papers everywhere. Liisa Kauppinen has become the new executive director of the Association.

I don't know any more how to sign in Finnish. Without noticing it I constantly use American signs. They now come to mind first. I'm ashamed; I've always laughed at people who spend a couple of years abroad and can't speak their mother tongue properly any more. Now I understand them better.

"You look sadder and more serious than before."

We sit in the Cellar Bar drinking coffee and eating Danish pastries. How awfully much they cost—everything here in the home country costs so much that no money seems to be enough, and I have to give up many items on my list. Liisa looks at me carefully; she is the only one who has time to come and chat with me. All the others act as if they have a fire under them. One hardly lifted her gaze from the typewriter, and yet everybody in their letters had told me how eagerly they waited for me to come and visit.

Sadder? Is that so? Is that how I've changed? But looking sad and serious isn't really a change. I've never been able to laugh anywhere except in the deaf world. Using sign language has always made me laugh and look happy. Liisa has

— 218 —

always seen me happy. And now I have my hearing-world expression on; it has stayed on because I haven't yet renewed my contact with this world where I can laugh.

From Liisankatu I walk to the Esplanadi in the gray afternoon; snow is drifting a little bit. I have tea with Rea Stadius in the Cafe Manta. Rea's father was one of the founding members of the Deaf Association at the turn of the century. I ponder how I can tell my friends what I've experienced in St. Lucia. The situation in St. Lucia is completely different from over here, and yet the problems of the deaf are basically the same everywhere.

When two weeks have passed, Jukka calls. Jukka misses me; he suggests that I might come home in only two more weeks. It depends on me whether I leave or not. And I feel that if I stay any longer, I can't leave at all; I'll become sick or something. Keke says that Father needs me more now than the boys do themselves. I can see that the boys are getting along fine. The whole house is waiting to get back to the everyday routines.

I leave. It's my birthday; tulips shine in vases, it's very cold outside. I turn forty on the plane.

I leave snowy, cold Finland where even the people seemed frozen—serious and stiff. But it's my own country, my roots are there. And the boys are there. No wonder I feel like crying when the plane swerves above the misty, frozen scenery. I wear a fur coat, woolen cap, mittens, scarf, and winter boots, and in my mind are memories of sauna, of talking with the boys, my sister-in-law Leena, my parents, mother-in-law, relatives. My father cried and said that he will miss me. He has never been ashamed of expressing his feelings.

Have I really been in Finland? It's like a dream.

Jukka meets me on the terrace, tanned. Instead of the dark and icy runway of my dream there is a yellow-green field surrounded by palms in the glow of the tropical sunset.

I am almost last to come out of the plane because my seat was in the rear of the plane. I have my fur coat in my arms and other winter garments in a plastic bag. I drag myself through the airport to customs. I know what Jukka is thinking: the little, tired cocker spaniel returning home with her tail between her legs. The journey was not what I expected, but it was good as it was. I saw the boys, and that was the main point.

"How wonderful to be back here again," I tell Jukka. "It's so warm and light, and the people—even they are warm and happy."

"But there is so much negative over here, too," Jukka reminds me.

Yes, if the journey has given me nothing else, at least it has brought my two home countries closer to each other, smoothed their differences. The island is no longer the exotic, wonderful place it was when we arrived almost two years ago. And there aren't so many things in my home country that I miss; they have partly lost their glow as well. Like toys I dreamed of during the war—they were left at home when we went to Granny's. By the time we came back after the war, I was a big girl. My toys were only a doll without a nose, a teddy bear who could turn his head, and blocks that could make many fairy tales. Dreaming of them was much better than getting them back, and yet they were dear.

Jeri and Alfonso are happy at my homecoming. The house smells of wetness and mosquito coil. It's the same kind of odor the books and papers have, curled up from dampness during the rainy season.

The house looks empty. Everything is clean and untouched because Jukka never leaves his things lying around.

Now that my traveling bags and presents are all topsy-turvy in the bedroom, the house starts to look as if somebody lives here.

Jukka makes tea and busies himself with the newspaper. He has kept the house in order for almost four weeks, fixed breakfast, kept Alfonso fed, taken Jeri out and fed him, taken Alfonso to school, done the grocery shopping, kept Zenia and Anderson in order.

We have tea together, and I tell him about the journey, of everything that it wasn't, and Jukka nods, satisfied: more proof that I can't get along without Jukka, as well as that Jukka needs me, too. Once we talked of the possibility of the other one's not being here any longer. Then one just would have to survive; there would be no alternative. After all the feelings of togetherness you owe it to the other one to get by alone, when faced with that situation.

We don't say anything about Jukka's new religious feelings, which he wrote to me about when I was in Finland. I am too embarrassed to talk about it, although I feel that I should say that I am happy for him and want to support him.

Several years ago, Keke gave his life to God at the church confirmation camp, and after that I often discussed God and life with him until midnight. At that time Jukka was busy evenings and weekends. He was head of Kotka's Hietanen Port organization project. I noticed that although I had believed in God since I was a little girl, I had not consciously considered the whole matter. Now I had to talk with Keke and read books, and I started to see things differently. Sometimes I also told Jukka about these thoughts. And now while he's been alone, Jukka has been reading and thinking, and he's made his decision to give his life to God. He has been affected most by words from Birgitta Yavari's book, *There's Love*:

> *What does it benefit a man*
> *if he with full sails*
> *in the fair wind*
> *of admiration and celebration*
> *roams the world*
> *but ends up on the beach of eternity*
> *a wreck?*

As it is written in the Bible:

"For what is a man profited, if he shall gain the whole world, and lose his own soul."

Maybe I'm confused because all of a sudden Jukka has gone further than I. I have to follow him over the threshold. Books and writings that were just phrases suddenly open up; it's as if we've found the key to them.

But now we just talk about Zenia and Alfonso and the island. I am thoroughly exhausted. One phase has ended and another has begun. But I have to rest now, from my cold dream in which there were still many spots of warmth. Actually, the whole journey was very important. It just wasn't what I planned it to be.

END OF STORY

Winter on the island is dry and sunny. It feels good to sit on the balcony, writing. There's no need even to go to the beach. In the afternoon it's easy to go to school in this refreshing weather. I enjoy walking slowly through the park to the schoolyard. Beyond the park the blooming tulip tree can be seen dimly. In the afternoons when I get home from school and Jukka returns from work, we go to the beach. Jeri swims long distances and fetches a stick; the hotel guests come and pat him and talk with us.

Alfonso is active and diligent. He has collected seeds from different trees and bushes. He makes beautiful bead necklaces that once again prove what an artistic eye he has. Seeds grouped by different colors and sizes become beautiful jewelry in his hands. Maybe Alfonso can earn his living by selling these necklaces to tourists.

Alfonso also washes the car, takes care of the garden, sweeps the stairs. Without grumbling, he does whatever Jukka asks him to do, although sometimes he complains that his wrists are sore from waxing the cars. But it will be good for Alfonso to learn to work. A couple of hours a day is not too much to demand. He is at school during the day; in the afternoons he goes to the beach to swim, to dig crabs, to jog.

Jukka takes responsibility for him. They have made contact and learned to communicate. I am happy that everything is going so well for Alfonso. It feels as if we've sailed into quiet waters after the storm. It's easier for me now that Jukka has taken so much responsibility for Alfonso. Less and less he says "Go and tell that boy" or "Go and look what that boy is doing downstairs."

When I went to school for the first time after my trip, they had the record player on and the children were dancing. I have come in the middle of carnival preparations—the annual great occasion on St. Lucia is getting close. First there will be the children's own carnivals in which our pupils will now also take part.

There on the wall are the postcards I sent from Finland. I chose the ones with the most snow, ice, and frozen weather in them. They look really exotic here.

"I didn't know there was so much snow in your home country!" Cynthia says.

Yet the amount of snow I saw back home was very modest compared to the amount the Canadian hotel guests were telling me about. In their country they sometimes have to dig the houses and cars out from under the snow. How about the United States this year of 1977—snow and below freezing temperatures even in regions that are usually warm. Even in Florida and the Bahamas it's cold. Suppose the climate of St. Lucia all of a sudden turned cold like that?

On Sunday we take Alfonso to the school. The children are being dressed up in carnival clothes: hearts, aces, spades, clubs, diamonds, kings, soldiers in red pants. Alfonso will be a diamond king. His first carnival! He has seen them before, of course—he stood in the street and mingled with the spectators, but was never really part of it, dancing and enjoying himself. We watch him being dressed. Somehow I feel that this day is a climax—Alfonso is nice and helpful, and so interested.

The children's carnivals are being held on the grounds of St. Mary's College. When the group from the school for the deaf is performing, Alfonso jumps clumsily, but he is in it, with the others performing!

I've forgotten all the difficulties we've had. It's such a long time ago . . . First there was Christmas, then I was sick, then I went back home. We've had no problems for two months. Alfonso is "our son," beautiful, happy, and cheerful.

However, on the evening of this fine and sunny day everything starts to go downhill for some reason. The visible reason is the bead necklaces Alfonso has made, but everything has to have been hidden somewhere much deeper, in our relationship with Alfonso and in his thoughts.

I don't know exactly what made me think about the bead necklaces that he had made just that morning. Before we left for the carnival I bought three necklaces for a dollar apiece. Alfonso put the money in a metal cigar box, but didn't take any money along to the carnival. When I told him that he could buy some sweets with it, Alfonso only shook his head laughing. He knew this, like many other things, so much better than I.

The question of money is a difficult one, and it becomes an insurmountable obstacle. We're not just being frugal by not giving Alfonso very much pocket money. We would only do him harm if we gave him too much of everything.

In the evening Alfonso asks me: "How much?"

He shows me the dollars he has put in the tin can, points to the bead necklaces hanging on the wall and to the beach. I realize that those three dollars are the start for Alfonso's business. He is asking me how much he could ask for the necklaces from the tourists on the beach.

But I haven't thought that Alfonso would earn money yet. It would make everything so much more complicated. It's hard for him to realize that his upkeep in general costs us something. He does understand poverty, but if he now has everything, he doesn't understand where it comes from. We have been planning to prepare Alfonso to earn his living when we're no longer here to look after him. We intend to arrange things, to set Alfonso's life in order before we leave to go back home. Jukka will look for a job for him, we'll give somebody the right to look after him and offer money. Alfonso will never be in need.

But that time has not yet come, and now he's starting too soon. Everything could go completely wrong. Alfonso might lose his chance. Maybe I'm wrong. Maybe he wouldn't even get his necklaces sold or would soon grow tired.

I will never know what way would have been the best one. The one I chose led to a conflict.

I try to explain the matter to him:

"Now you learn how to make necklaces. You learn which seeds are the best and will last. You won't sell anything yet. I give you food and clothes and room. Later I go away. Then you sell necklaces and get money and buy food and clothes yourself." I explain how Alfonso then will have to pay for his room, electricity, everything. I can see that the boy doesn't understand. I explain and explain, but finally I feel that Jukka's forefinger is needed.

Jukka comes, and the forefinger speaks. The finger points to the necklaces and the nail: "The necklaces will stay there."

That's all.

Alfonso understands. The necklaces stay on the wall. But Alfonso doesn't understand why.

Lying in bed that night, I decided that I have to teach Alfonso that food for him doesn't come like manna from heaven. I decide that next morning Alfonso won't get his breakfast until he has swept the stairs. I help him by giving him food. He helps me by sweeping the stairs. There's no money needed from either party. Everyone in the family does his duties.

In the morning when I open the kitchen door I can see that Alfonso looks defiant. I should leave him be and think it over. But no, I'm too concerned over his attitude and too hasty in trying to change it. I have to make him understand. Right now.

I push the broom into his hand. I explain all that I have thought through about helping each other, with no money needed from either side. Alfonso will now sweep the stairs, and I will prepare the breakfast tray.

Alfonso doesn't take the broom; he hangs his head and looks sullen. I wait for a while. I take the broom again and try again. He has got to understand. It is important. I have to win in this matter.

But Alfonso does something that I never expected, although I should have guessed it from his defiant eyes. Yesterday's happy day is still too near. Was it only yesterday?

Alfonso goes to the dining room and tears the picture he has made in school from the wall, the picture he had given me after I asked for it. He doesn't seem to understand that gifts are not taken away.

"Let the picture be."

We are pulling at the picture between us. I wish Jukka were here to tell him that the picture will stay where it is now.

Of course Alfonso is stronger, and anger doubles his strength. He goes downstairs with determined steps, the picture under his arm. To pack? It looks like it. What happens is what I've been unconsciously expecting the whole time, and at some difficult moments even wished for: Alfonso packs and leaves.

Well, let him go. He can pack and leave.

But after a while something inside of me says that I can't give up.

I go downstairs. He has packed all his things in plastic bags and boxes.

I pick up scissors, tubes of glue, and sewing equipment out of a box.

"These things are not yours!"

Alfonso drags everything back, and for a while we scuffle.

"They are mine. Mine. I have swept, washed the car. I haven't received any salary. I will take these for my salary."

Alfonso is gesturing wildly, full of rage.

Is that so? How long has Alfonso nourished this defiance in his mind, that he hasn't been paid for washing the car or sweeping the stairs?

I try to explain for the last time.

That Jukka and I have paid for the electricity, room, food, clothes, everything. Alfonso has got money for movies. A two-hour job isn't enough to pay for all this, but we have given this all to Alfonso for love, as if to our own child. We only demand the same as parents demand of their child. We have wanted to teach him to work. Anderson could just as well have washed the car, and it's Zenia's duty to sweep the stairs.

I pick up the things that are not his. We fight, moving all around the room. Finally Alfonso yells. He bursts out with unintelligible sounds in a rough voice from his throat—they mean something in his mind, but they don't tell me anything but that he's violently angry. His face is contorted, red with rage.

Instinctively I change my approach. Alfonso knows God and heaven, they have been discussed in school, and Alfonso has gone to church like all islanders.

"God in heaven can see what you are doing. You're doing wrong. I have loved you like my own son. Who will love you in the mountains and in town if you leave?"

This is true. Alfonso will not find love anywhere. I have really wanted to love this child as my own, although I haven't always succeeded in doing so. Elsewhere he will only face discrimination, I know that for certain.

Maybe it's easier for Alfonso to understand hatred!

I am humble in front of him. I have fought, raged, spoken wisely, threatened, become humble. Nothing seems to help. Alfonso is so full of defiance and aggression that it's bursting out of him. His eyes are bulging out of his head; he's actually choking with rage.

I give up. I can't do anything. He can go.

"Let him go then; it can't be helped. Calm down," Jukka says when he comes home for lunch. But I can't calm down. I feel ashamed that I became humble in front of Alfonso, that I talked about love and God. Humbling myself in front of that young colt who has behaved shamelessly toward me. Would I feel any better if I had thrown his boxes and plastic bags out and the boy after them?

In the afternoon I watch out of the corner of my eye as Alfonso walks along the road. He comes from the beach, has all of a sudden changed his clothes, and is going to town. His things are somewhere, hidden under the bushes.

Poor boy, doesn't he know what he wants? Doesn't he have a place to stay? I can see how he looks defiantly toward our house. Maybe he hopes I'll run after him and ask him to come back. But I won't do it.

The boy hasn't eaten anything, but he has been hungry before. It's not enough to make him change his mind.

Finally Alfonso goes to town. During the carnival week there has been something happening all the time. Steel bands and singers are competing the whole week on the Square and in the park; people are dancing in the street.

I sleep badly. In my dreams I expect a knock on the door, the furious banging of Alfonso's fists, the tired and hungry boy outside the door. But nothing happens . . . until five o'clock in the morning.

Jeri barks. Alfonso has come back. I am so exhausted that I stay in bed. Jukka takes care of it.

An hour later Jukka comes back to the bedroom, and I learn what has happened.

Alfonso is now in his room. Five policemen have brought him! The boy had been returning home (home!). He'd been in town all night. Somewhere along the way, somebody mistook him for a cow thief. Maybe he milked a cow in his hunger, but what sense would there have been in stealing a cow!

Alfonso got caught, the police were called, and five men appeared. The boy was asked where he lived, and he guided the police to our house.

"Does this boy live here? He was caught stealing a cow."

"Yes, he lived with us, but this afternoon he packed his things and left."

When faced with superior power, Alfonso shows where his things are. The boxes are brought from under the bush into his room. Jukka's forefinger speaks: things will be sorted out into two piles. This is Alfonso's, that, ours.

In principle, Alfonso has committed theft. He has taken away things that are not his own.

"Do you want us to take the boy to the police station?"

"No, the boy can stay if he wants."

Now the police are gone. I go to see Alfonso. He sits in his room in the middle of his things and looks exhausted. But his defiance and aggressiveness have not diminished one bit.

"You can stay or leave. You unpack your things, and I bring breakfast."

"I go away."

"Where would you go?"

"To mother. Here I work and don't get paid."

Peter Paul comes in the afternoon and tries to talk some sense into Alfonso.

"Won't you thank Raija and Jukka?"

"No need to thank." Alfonso makes a belittling gesture and swings his hand again towards the stairs. "I have swept and washed the car, and not got money."

"He can go then," I say, feeling weary. "Take him to his mother when he's ready to leave."

First I bring him a tray—he doesn't need to leave hungry.

I have never before seen him with such a victorious smile as now, when he is biting into the toast.

I get his things from downstairs.

Peter Paul takes them. Alfonso follows him to the car. He doesn't even look at me. The car drives away. Peter Paul does so much for us!

In the evening I ask Jukka where Peter Paul took Alfonso.

"He is staying at Peter Paul's house now."

Peter Paul drove Alfonso around the island for the whole day.

First to his mother in the Rainforest Village. She has a flock of children, too many mouths to feed. Besides, Grandmother adopted the boy when he was a baby.

They drive to the grandmother.

"I can't take, bad boy."

They go to the uncle.

"Can't take."

None of the relatives wants Alfonso. Stupid boy; why didn't he stay where he was given food and clothes!

Poor boy. He doesn't have a place to go. It's easy to be defiant and leave—

it's a completely different matter to find a roof over one's head and money for living.

Alfonso sits apathetically in the car. Peter Paul drives around in town and finally they go to the harbor office.

Jukka calls up Cornell, whom he always asks for advice. What to do? How far does our responsibility for the boy reach? Suppose we let him stay?

Cornell offers the advice that we can take the boy to the social authorities. There's no point in us continuing with the boy, or so it appears.

There are social authorities on the island, but there's not much they can do, because they don't have the means. The streets are filled with homeless children who go from one relative to another and beg on the street during the day. The social authorities take over and promise to find Alfonso a place, if nothing else at least in a center for homeless boys.

Now Alfonso is at Peter Paul's, in any case. Peter Paul takes him to see the carnival procession with his own children.

We also go to see the procession. In the sunny streets where people dressed in their best, eagerly crowding together waiting for the procession, I forget Alfonso. Somewhere in the midst of umbrellas, brightly dressed people, and ice cream sellers, he stretches on tiptoe to see, with Peter's children. Maybe he also forgets the unpleasantness and enjoys the procession with its color, rhythm, and cheerfulness.

Of course the procession lets us wait for it; nothing here on the island starts punctually—but the spectators have come early to reserve the best places along the Boulevard and the streets near it where the view is best.

People along the streets are waiting, chewing candy, nuts, and ice cream bought from the sellers on the streets. Sometimes it rains, sometimes the sun is shining—the umbrella helps in both cases.

We go to the Islander Club by the Boulevard; we pay the entrance fee, climb up to the terrace and wait.

From the eager and waiting uproar I know when the first group is getting close. I see a colorful mass that sways back and forth. In front, a truck carries two tiers of steel bands drumming on halves of barrels. The players drum rhythmically, and the truck platform sways with the rhythm.

Then come figures in imaginative costumes. They move from the bottom of their hearts. The rhythm spreads; the crowd gets caught up in it and feels the same foaming cheerfulness as those who dance on the street. It reminds me of a march; the same tempo and beat repeat themselves endlessly. So much color and rhythm slides past us that it's almost too much. And when the last group has passed us, the whole crowd from along the streets joins in and unloads all the energy they've felt as they watched the dancers and swayed in time with them. The streets are full of dancers for hours.

By the post office we see George and Merle dancing in the middle of the crowd. We're pulled along—we dance along Bridge Street and turn onto Jeremie Street, near the harbor and the marketplace. People keep following the steel band truck like the Pied Piper in the fairy tale. We dance until we're gasping. A great time! We feel like St. Lucians today!

The next day Peter Paul drives me shopping. He tells me that the social authorities have found a family of relatives who will take Alfonso in.

"Alfonso was sad."

"Yes, maybe later on he can come back to us."

But can he? I don't believe it. My heart is close to breaking, but at the same time I'm relieved, as if a burden had been lifted from me. Maybe I wasn't mature enough to carry it, or maybe the task was impossible to start with, although there was good will and willingness to help. Maybe I didn't have enough love, or maybe—however unconsciously—I expected to get thanks for a good deed. I don't know.

But I can't help it that I breathe more freely, enjoy the beautiful, sunny winter so much. I try to tell myself that I can't take this incident too seriously. I couldn't help it. And I feel that I don't have the energy to take Alfonso back again.

We have had time to affect him somewhat. He isn't the same lonely savage that he was seven months ago. He doesn't necessarily need to be isolated and rejected—he has acquaintances now with whom he can communicate. He will never again sink down to the level of the boy from the fish market.

Jukka says that there's no need for us to explain to people how and why Alfonso left. Jukka is always so careful in his speech. There's no need to tell something that's unnecessary and could cause misunderstanding. One never knows how people will react. The locals often take each other's side.

I can't help talking about the matter, though, because I feel that I've been judged wrongly, and the bitterness has to be eased. It was I who gave the boy food and home, and what did I get for it? Kenneth and Victor tell me eagerly that they are willing to come to live in Roger's room, willing to wash the car and do anything.

Kenneth complains constantly that he doesn't get food, and that he is beaten, always pushed from one relative to another. I can't completely believe him; he doesn't look as if he's in need, but he begs constantly. That's why I don't give him anything. Victor never begs, although he must be hungry sometimes. Joseph has a home, food, and love; he is strongly built, a well-balanced boy.

Alfonso doesn't come to school; but some of the boys have seen him in town, and Alfonso has told them that he has "skedaddled" and "doesn't care about Raija." Both of these expressions require only a single gesture that communicates much better than any words. These gestures go through my heart like a dagger. Maybe intonation can affect hearing people in the same way.

The boys think that Alfonso is stupid. And in the sunny yard, small children circle around me.

"Roger? Raija? Home?"

"Roger away. Roger wants to leave. Does not want food and home," I sign to the children.

The children look at me with round, wondering eyes. I don't understand why they have always been so interested in Alfonso's living with us.

One afternoon when I step into the classroom, my heart shrinks. Alfonso is sitting at the table doing woodwork.

"Roger is here," Kenneth and Joseph are signing.

I shrug my shoulders. Is that so! I don't even look at the boy; I'm angry. From one afternoon to another I don't say anything and don't look toward Alfonso, and he pretends not to see me. Sometimes when I look at him by chance I can see that his eyes are endlessly sad, but yet defiant.

Sometimes Alfonso passes Jukka and me when we go to the beach. The boy hurries by us with his cap tightly over his head, looking dark and angry; it is as if he is darkened by his anger.

Does he detest me so much? I try to look calm.

But in school Alfonso's appearance is tired and sad. He must understand that he has lost something. His clothes are dirtier and dirtier, and he comes to school only rarely.

Most of the time he sits all day long as if in a daze in front of the M. K. C. department store near the fruit stalls. He stares at the mangoes, bananas, and candy on the table, at the boy with cerebral palsy who sits in his wheelchair under the store roof, and at people who walk by in an endless stream. Alfonso stares for hours without really seeing anything, doing nothing, sunken into idleness.

And yet those hands are strong and skillful; they could produce a lot, his brains have the capacity for learning. So much is wasted. Something went wrong, and I don't know why.

But there are still others whose hands and minds I can help to develop. I'm in a hurry. Our pupils finish their schooling this year. Maybe they will go to work before school ends. Clyde's two-year term is getting close to the end; he is counting the months, weeks, days. It has been hard for him in many ways. Two years ago he got a group of completely wild children who had to be collected from the parks and streets into the classroom. Luckily, Clyde had enough authority and ability to handle them, otherwise nothing would have come of it.

Now his class has formed into something completely different—more social, more mature. But Clyde has needed much more help than I've been able to give him. Maybe Clyde is tired of what also tires me: that everything is still so vague. Frameworks and systems haven't been created for the school. They will be created later on; they are forming already, but everything happens so slowly here. Somebody has to lay the foundation. For my own part I can at least be proud of the fact that I have worked at the school for a year and a half. Other volunteer helpers have come and gone; I haven't given up.

I know all the pupils love Clyde. They are already grieving that in a couple of months Clyde will fly fa-fa-fa home to America. It's hard for them to understand it completely, but they talk about it and feel sorry.

And I know well that Clyde loves "his children"—he speaks all the time of "my children," and I'm a bit jealous, because in my opinion the children are partly mine, too. I think "my girls," because I'm worried about the girls, what they will learn, what they will become, how they'll get by.

Of course Clyde often gets angry at the young people and yells at them. He is tired and frustrated; the pupils make noise, are unattentive, don't want to learn. But it's better than if he tried to be patient and sweet all the time. In their environment the deaf young people have to get used to the whole scale of emotions. They don't hear the intonation, but they understand gestures and facial expressions. I remember how, in the beginning, I saw Clyde's behavior toward the children as too harsh.

Clyde is worried about what the youngsters will do after he leaves. I assure him that I'll take care of them as long as I'm on the island. But of course it would be nicer in Clyde's opinion to think that he's irreplaceable, and I won't say anything any more.

But I also long for the feeling of being needed, the feeling that I've done something good. Clyde has never noticed that.

I think to myself how I would arrange some activity after Clyde is gone. In some way the youngsters have to feel that I am available if they need help, and they should be able to get together in some kind of a club, a Deaf Club. It's Clyde's goal to arrange jobs for all the children before he leaves.

We are doing handiwork at full force with the girls, but how can I get them to concentrate, to turn their eyes away from whatever is happening on the boys' side or in the park? Theresa turns her head obediently, but I have to tap Magilda and finally pull at her chin to get her head to turn. Even then her eyes and thoughts are still on what she has seen in the park.

Magilda is not the shy and quiet girl I took her for in the beginning. She learned sign language fast, and now that she has learned to communicate, she's lively and spirited. She wears her hair in two thick braids, and she has tennis shoes on her feet, but she's growing out of them, ripening right in front of our eyes. And when she comes to school with her hair in a round knot, she looks more mature than her age.

One day I see that Magilda is standing in the yard looking fierce, feet apart, with her fists ready to lash out. Standing opposite her is a hearing schoolgirl who was standing in the classroom door this morning, staring at us.

The sight makes me laugh, although I understand that there's nothing to laugh about. The fights between women on the island are violent and unpreventable—there's no room for mercy.

"Go away. There's no fighting in the schoolyard," says Clyde.

The girls leave the yard, but I can see that they intend to fight in the park; the conflict has to be cleared up. In her anger, Magilda has pushed the other girl, and now the girl wants retribution.

But nothing comes of the fight. I watch with surprise as Kenneth, Joseph, and Victor step in between them! Last year they would have stirred up the fight, but now they want to make sure that nothing bad happens to Magilda, who is one of them!

When I go to town shopping after school in the afternoons I can see the whole class loafing around in the streets together. It warms my heart; the children have found each other. Only Filipa is an outsider, too much in her own world.

To my surprise Clyde informs me, glowing with satisfaction: "I have good news. The girls have jobs as seamstresses at 'My Fair'."

I am quite astonished. How on earth has it been possible to find jobs for the girls just like that on an island where unemployment is high and where so little is known of deafness?

Clyde met the manager of My Fair at a party, pulled out his pen and paper, and got the manager interested in him. The discussion turned to the school and to the deaf girls who don't have jobs. And the manager is interested in everything: he even wants to study sign language!

"You go with the girls to the factory during their training period," Clyde says. "You get to be in an air-conditioned room," he adds proudly.

So that's how we girls have a month now to finish all our courses in handicraft and cooking and to learn everything connected with work: "Dear girls, when you go to work you can't stare out the window the whole time and sign to each other. You have to tramp on the sewing machine treadle without a break. And sit up with your back straight; start right now. Theresa, if you sit like that the whole time, you'll get a sore back soon and won't be able to sew any more."

I ponder how Theresa will get by at work. She seems to get tired just during the school day, which is much shorter than a working day.

It doesn't take long for Clyde to inform us that he has found jobs for Kenneth and Joseph, too. They were accepted by Ferrand's Dairy to make ice cream and milk out of powder. So now four youngsters have jobs already. Valerie can't go to the clothing factory because of her bad eyesight; we don't know about

Filipa yet. We have doubts about her ability to work—she might learn to sew, but would she go to the factory every day on time, and would she understand how to follow all the rules?

Alfonso comes to school very rarely, but Clyde arranges for him and Victor to be at a boys' craft workshop. They won't get much of a salary, but it will be good practice. And later on we can try to find them better jobs. Poor Alfonso! Jukka could have found him a really good job!

One day I take the girls to the beach and tell them we're going to have a whole day of physical exercise and sports. I show them exercises to strengthen their back muscles so their backs won't get tired at the sewing machine. When we visited the factory I noticed that the chairs didn't fulfill any ergonomic demands at all. The factory hall is air-conditioned, but the chairs are from the Middle Ages!

The girls romp and splash in the water and spatter water on each other. Nobody can swim. I teach every one in turn, but then they notice a mango tree on shore, and in a minute Magilda is in the tree dropping fruit to the ground. Greenish mangoes plop on the ground and in the water; we pick them up, racing one another. I sit with the girls on the beach sucking mangoes. Picked straight from the tree and eaten on the beach they taste delicious, and after that I am a mango lover.

"Look here, now we'll exercise." I show the girls movements, and they try to do the same, but they aren't able to do even the simplest movement. Their coordination is clumsy, like that of small children. I feel agile compared to them, although their figures are as slim as willow branches compared to me. Sometimes in their straightforward manner the girls show me how wide my backside is. Sometimes I explain how women in my country have much wider hips than women on the island. Although I must admit I have gained some weight on the island—quite a lot. I love the pumpkin soups, christophene au gratin, fried plantains, breadfruit casseroles, crabs, rotis, fishballs. There are just too many parties with sagging tables.

I dig into my basket and get rolls and a big thermos of coffee for the girls. Coffee is a part of my life in every situation, and these girls drink it now, too, with a lot of sugar and milk in it.

Then we go to our house, and the girls go to the shower screaming and giggling and comb their hair with long-toothed combs. When they're ready, they ask me to take a photo of them. Of course Jeri gets in the picture—he's always in the picture somehow.

Theresa stays with us all evening. She sits in the living room and looks through all my photo albums. In one album there are photos of my relatives, godchildren, and closest friends. I have noticed before how interested the deaf children are in our photos.

Clyde has also decided to give his last finishing touches to the upbringing of the girls. One afternoon when I enter the classroom I see that Magilda sits at the end of the long table and beats on the typewriter with uncertain strokes like someone who has just started to experiment with it. Theresa sits besides her and cries bitterly. Clyde is furious.

Clyde has tried to teach typewriting to Theresa, and Theresa, as usual, has just looked around helplessly. She doesn't have the self-confidence to reach out her finger and strike a key. The whole machine frightens her.

I feel sorry for the girl; she cries so pitifully. I can understand how she feels. Haven't I been uncertain so often when faced with something new, not daring to get started, not daring to trust myself to do this strange thing?

But Clyde is too angry. How does shouting help when a person is in the trough of the wave? I tap Theresa on the shoulder and give her a handkerchief.

"Do wash your face, don't cry any more."

Maybe it will happen to Theresa as it has happened to me so many times. After calming down she may think about the matter differently and learn from it that one should not give in, one should keep trying. That's how things start working. And if something goes wrong, it doesn't stop the world from going around.

Clyde explains that these youngsters should understand their deafness and the problems it causes, but these young people think it doesn't matter that they are deaf.

"I have studied and gone forward, become conscious of my problems and purposefully triumphed over them. In America the deaf people learn, and they talk about their problems, but these young people here don't want to learn anything."

Well, Clyde is tired and impatient. You can't compare America and St. Lucia. His pupils are the first deaf people in St. Lucia who have ever gone to school, and they are now finishing school after only two years. It's only a very small start at becoming conscious of problems, talking about them, and getting rid of them.

It's empty in the classroom. The boys have started their work at the dairy and the workshop. Clyde is with them; I finish handicrafts with the girls. They're sewing handkerchiefs by hand now. A thin needle can stay steady in their fingers, and the stitches are pretty. I wanted to teach them to sew on a sewing machine, but there's no time, and we have no machine at school. The girls have learned what they've been able to learn.

We've had a crafts exhibition. Out in the park two tables were set up, one for the girls to show their work, the other one for the boys. Each table is beautiful and colorful. It's a pity that nobody will see them, because the whole thing is only for Clyde to photograph. Of course he wants photos of his achievements. I notice that my achievements are also his achievements. I already have a picture where I stand behind the handiwork table with Theresa, Magilda, Filipa, and Valerie beside me. My girls.

The boys learn how to use the ice cream machines at the dairy. They come to the school during lunch hour to see the girls and to show them what they do. You stamp on this and press that and pull. I'm reminded of the time the Theatre of the Deaf staged a Swedish play that featured a pantomime sketch of factory work.

Clyde arranges union membership cards for the girls and drops in to tell us how the boys are doing in their work.

Finally, there is the last school day, even for the girls. The boys come and ·visit during the lunch hour. I have never before sensed such a friendship between these youngsters as now, when they all suddenly realize that their school days are over, that everything from now on will be different from what it has been before. All squabbles are over, only the nice moments are remembered.

The boys wave sadly from the door. Kenneth crosses his arms on his breast: *love.*

Clyde has had dinner with the manager of My Fair and taught him fifty signs. The manager is exceptionally interested. I understand it: when the right person is talking about it, the deaf world is an extraordinarily interesting new world.

MY FAIR

The practice period at My Fair begins. In the mornings I meet the girls at the factory gate. I explain over and over that they shouldn't be late, because for three late arrivals one is fired without appeal. We put our things in the locker, stamp our time cards, go to the cool hall where women talk to each other beside their machines before they begin treadling vigorously.

There is already one deaf young woman, Arlette, in the factory. Arlette works neatly and diligently, sitting with a straight back. She is the embodiment of a good worker. That kind will always help other deaf people get jobs.

I have met Arlette already, visiting her home with Clyde. Arlette has a deaf sister, Kathleen, and two deaf brothers. Both girls are nice and seem sensible. They have not been at school at all, but they have an exceptionally wise mother who has been able to guide her daughters. The girls are fashionably dressed, pretty and well-combed, also well-behaved. The boys are more reserved. The mother and the children have developed their own sign language, but now Arlette, Theresa, and Magilda understand each other completely.

I regret that we didn't have sewing machines at school. Then the girls wouldn't have so much to learn now. Theresa and Magilda treadle their machines in an unskilled rhythm; the needles tick too fast, go everywhere and break. Again we have to ask the boy to repair it. The women around them are laughing; they sew without trouble and diligently, their movements light and soft (like those of all the other people here, not like my movements, heavy and slow).

Arlette shows the girls how to do it. Her foot treadles gracefully, pushing along just the right amount at the right time. The needle ticks smoothly and accurately, stops just where it should, and doesn't go on its own way, wherever.

The thread stays in its place, and the needle doesn't break. And if the thread does slip away, she can put it back in its place even in her sleep.

Magilda and Theresa do not yet remember the complicated procedure of passing the thread through from spool to needle.

Arlette opens her hands like a magician who has performed a difficult trick without trouble. She shrugs her shoulders. "Look here, it's not difficult at all!"

Suppose I myself had to sew these small pieces into their proper place? I wouldn't do any better. It's good that we have Arlette here, preventing my ignorance from being revealed!

The machines crackle, and there must be music somewhere, because the girls who examine and pack finished T-shirts are swaying and taking dancing steps once in a while. I turn off my hearing aid for proof and am surprised at the change that occurs in the whole scene. The ticking of the needles and the crackle of dozens of sewing machines at the same time make the factory hall seem busy; without sound the whole sense of diligence is gone. There's no rhythm to follow. The deaf girls have to create their own rhythm, each feeling only the vibration of her own machine.

How do they experience and interpret the mouths that open to say a word to somebody close by or spread into a laugh when once again Magilda's needle breaks? How do they interpret all those eyes that sometimes turn toward them— curious or amused, friendly or hostile, sympathetic or indifferent? But the glances are brief. You aren't allowed to look around or chat; you have to work. The boss comes once in a while to check; he's patient, saying that all the girls have had difficulties in the beginning. He taps us all encouragingly on the shoulders and continues on his way.

The morning goes by slowly, but finally it's ten o'clock. The women are pushing in a crowd to stamp their cards, and to my great surprise there's somebody to advise the girls. In all that laughing group there is, in fact, sympathy toward these deaf girls, which promises well. Clearly, Arlette seems to be happy that she finally has deaf co-workers. And although the girls are sitting separate from the others, there's no gap between them and the hearing girls. The girls are one with this group, sitting on benches in a gloomy dining room, drinking coffee or Pepsi, and sucking mangoes.

Theresa and Magilda have with them only a couple of rolls and bottles of red soft drink; how will this give them strength for the day's work? But I know these girls well. I have with me in my bag a big bottle of coffee with a lot of cream and sugar, and a big pile of sandwiches with cheese and egg. I am like a mother hen to the girls. They lean on me just as at school. Now I have to support them so that they won't get frightened of their strange surroundings during these first days. But in a couple of weeks they will have to get along alone.

"Tomorrow, here, too?" Theresa asks with round eyes.

"Yes. And tomorrow-tomorrow and tomorrow-tomorrow-tomorrow. Next week, next month, and next year. If you learn well and work well."

The factory loses about ten needles a day during the following days, as well as both Arlette's and one repairman's share of the work. The director is beginning to be a bit impatient, but he still has hope. He has decided to employ these deaf girls.

"Magilda sick," Magilda complains on a couple of mornings. The boss brings pain relievers, but of course it doesn't help. Magilda has a headache because she hasn't eaten anything in the morning before coming to work.

"In the morning you eat well. And take along a dish full of food. Look. The other women have a dish of rice and fish or a bottle of soup. You have to eat so you have the strength to sew for the whole day."

I still have a bag of food with me, but again and again I explain to the girls that soon I won't come with them to the factory any more; they'll have to bring their own lunchboxes along. I can bring them coffee and sandwiches once in a while but not every day.

It's hard for the girls to understand that Raija won't be coming with them any more. Raija has been with them at school almost every day, hasn't she? Why won't she also be here now? Why doesn't Raija sew? Why doesn't she have her own yellow card and her own locker?

And I have to stop coming soon. Theresa won't ever learn to work and stand on her own feet if I'm there always sitting beside her. She shouldn't always ask for my approval with her glance. She has to approve or disapprove of herself, to decide for herself what she's going to do.

More and more often Arlette snaps forward the circle formed by her thumb and finger. Good! The girls are starting to learn, aren't they? There are days when not a single needle is broken, and Magilda already finishes a whole pile of underwear, its front and back halves neatly sewn together. There has been a lot of undoing, too, but somethings gets finished, and even Arlette gets her own full share done again. Magilda puts the day's numbers on the bonus list that is written at the end of every workday.

The director says that Theresa has also progressed, but she looks around too much and is very slow. She still has a couple of months of practice time left; maybe she'll learn.

I tell Theresa that she shouldn't keep glancing around. She has to sew the whole time, and only during breaks can she talk to Magilda and Arlette. That's all I can do. After two weeks I stay at home and hope for the best. Once in a while I visit the girls, take a bottle of coffee to them, wait until it's ten o'clock and they come out of the factory hall. Magilda already has a dish of food for lunch. Theresa still has only two rolls, and hunger will force her to take lunch along with her, if I don't bring her anything any more.

WEDNESDAY CLUB

I wait for the girls at four-thirty at the factory crossing. Clyde's departure is inescapably facing us. He has sent applications to the schools for the deaf in the United States. I wrote him a letter of recommendation in which I praised his ability to deal with his pupils. I wrote about how much they have progressed, considering how difficult the circumstances were, especially in the beginning.

But at the end Clyde has decided to go to Sierra Leone in Africa to spend two more years in a developing country. In Sierra Leone it will be Clyde's job to initiate the organizational activities of the deaf. The offer is tempting—two more years, and after that Clyde may go back home. Clyde's mother hopes that he will come home and get married.

Now we have a farewell party for Clyde at school. How many farewell parties have we on the island? There's always somebody leaving or arriving; you get used to it. A new teacher, Millie Brother, has already come to take Clyde's place. Millie is a hearing child of deaf parents, originally from California like Clyde.

The small children's classroom has been decorated, made into a festive hall. There's a tablecloth on the table and a colorful bouquet; the small back room is full of service trays and presents. The boys come from the dairy; some of the children's parents and members of the society are there, too. We sit and eat sandwiches, cakes, and candy; we drink juice, have speeches, give presents. Finally I push Clyde's present from our class into Kenneth's hands. The present is a pillow on which every pupil has sewn his own name with red thread. Kenneth has cut a big red heart and the letters L-O-V-E out of red material and sewn them on the pillow.

Kenneth goes and hands the pillow to Clyde, is bashful, signs simply "love." This releases the sadness and longing that is dammed up in Clyde. He weeps and embraces his "children"—"my children." He has to cut the ties that link him to the children. If everything had been easier, it would also have been easier to cut the ties and leave. But the ties are so strong because they have lasted without breaking through the troublesome, wild, molding process; they have been woven out of all that wearying work that wasn't seen. And even what could be seen—nobody can guess how much hard work was behind it all.

Maybe I'm the only one who really knows what Clyde has done or left undone, how many ideas he has had and how few opportunities he has had to realize them. But he truly can leave the island with a good conscience. If only he believed that I will take care of "his children"—but that's something he doesn't want to believe because it's nicer to think that he is irreplaceable. I hope that Clyde will have a good time in Africa—there, at least, there should be adult deaf people who know how to sign the way Clyde does.

How will I take care of "Clyde's children"? I have to think about that. But now it's already the end of May, and finally Keke and Joppe are coming back for their vacation. How many times have Jukka and I sat on the balcony, not knowing what to do with ourselves. In the evenings the darkness of the tropics surrounds us, the coils smelling, fireflies sparkling. Later on I will certainly miss these warm, soft evenings. In Finland it seems as if the immobile birches in the yard soar endlessly high, and the sky is far away, unreachable. Here the constantly moving tops of the palms and the colorful sky seem to be near, and nothing is ever completely immobile and quiet.

Before I have time to plan or organize anything, before I have time to decide where we would get together and when, the matter solves itself.

At sunset there's Kenneth, or Theresa, or Joseph, Magilda, or Arlette walking along the road, sometimes alone, sometimes two together, sometimes all of them together. They sit on the balcony with us for an hour, until the sun is so low that they have to start getting back home. I serve something to drink, cookies, sandwiches, soup, whatever I happen to have. I learn how everything is going at work, and I tell them whether I've seen other youngsters and how they're doing.

Finally I tell them that they all could come on Wednesdays, when I know I'll be at home. That way they'll get to see one another.

Sometimes I arrange a party for the young people: a lot of good food, dancing, a lot of signing. The most important thing is that the young people can be together. Maybe they can tell each other about their problems and the things that happen to them that my sign language skills don't quite cover. Magilda comes rarely. Everything goes well for her at work; she has hearing friends and she speaks quite understandably. She gets by with hearing people somehow. I imagine she might be in the same borderland as I, but doesn't realize yet that life is at its best when you know where you belong, when you can converse with complete freedom and always know what the other person means.

Each week I ask the girls how much they have sewn and Magilda lifts up more and more fingers. Three, four, five, six stacks she has tied together, and she has glued as many slips on her working sheet.

How about the salary? The manager gave out one violet, two green, and two red banknotes on Friday. Magilda has given a part of it to her aunt, and the aunt has bought a thermos bottle.

"Blue one," Magilda says proudly.

Theresa still sews only two stacks. And it doesn't take long till the manager asks to see me. Theresa doesn't progress at all; she knows now how to sew, but slowly. Her speed doesn't increase at all. Two stacks a day is too little. Arlette sews ten or more. The manager is sorry, but if Theresa doesn't sew faster after the trial period, she'll have to leave. It's the same with all the girls.

Next time Theresa comes I have a word with her. I cut slips out of paper and show how Theresa is sewing now. Slowly, taking her time and glancing around. Only two slips are glued on paper. But the manager is not satisfied. I show Theresa what the manager wants. I act out sewing in a blazing rush with my imaginary sewing machine, one stack after another, without glancing around, one, two, three, four stacks. More and more. Magilda sews six stacks, Arlette ten. Theresa sewed two yesterday, today two. Tomorrow and tomorrow-tomorrow two is not enough, but instead Theresa must stay at home.

"You like work?"

Theresa's fist and head move in the sign of agreement.

"Remember now, tomorrow you try to sew three stacks. You don't glance around; you just sew. Fast, fast, fast."

I don't know if Theresa will learn to sew faster. The problem is solved simply by the fact that a new factory manager takes over, and Theresa gets extra time. The new manager probably doesn't know of the warning she has had.

When I visit the factory to check on the situation, the manager is entirely happy. The deaf girls are magnificent workers; he is willing to take on even more of them.

A couple of times even Alfonso comes to the Wednesday Club. Smiling, and not completely forgotten. He seems at home, he knows the place.

It's Roger's pictures that Raija shows. Again we take the photos out, or the picture in the history book, the picture in which a fierce-looking white man carries a black girl through the jungle. The girl has an iron ring around her throat, a long chain hanging from it. I've wondered why that picture interests Alfonso so much. Does he guess that that's where his roots are? His foremothers and forefathers have been carried the same way in chains through the jungle and over the ocean—his and Joseph's and Kenneth's and Victor's ancestors. I sign that this all happened fa-fa-fa, a long time ago. But Alfonso sees that the woman is black like him and that there's despair in her eyes, like the sadness that often shows in his own eyes.

Alfonso doesn't stay long at the crafts workshop. Victor tells me that Alfonso comes to work whenever he wants. Sometimes I see Alfonso walking on the beach in the middle of the working day. I ask him why he isn't at the workshop.

"Tomorrow I will go," Alfonso confidently assures me. But tomorrow again it's nice to get up whenever he wants, go to the beach, to stay there as long as he wants, to catch fish for dinner.

One Wednesday Victor tells me that Alfonso has started to sell ice cream. He has a cart together with a hearing boy, and the boys are building a "house" in the mountains behind the town.

I guess Alfonso might be a salesman by nature. He can't be forced into any shape except the one he creates for himself. He doesn't know about anything beyond St. Lucia, but the other youngsters have learned more, and they suffer the pain of knowing. Somewhere far away there are countries where everything is better. Many men from St. Lucia have left. Of course they're doing fine, they have money and cars, they have something in their lives that Kenneth and Joseph don't quite grasp, but it's real, it's something good.

"St. Lucia bad. Fly away. To Canada and America," Kenneth says more and more often.

"No, St. Lucia is not bad. St. Lucia is good. Better than New York and London." I say this convincingly because I really think so. For these boys St. Lucia *is* better, if they don't go to a vocational school for the deaf somewhere abroad to continue their studies.

I don't know how this dissatisfaction has spread to the boys. Before, they didn't know that there was a world beyond St. Lucia. Maybe it feels good to Kenneth and Joseph to have this idea that they can get away, when standing in the hot dairy by the ice cream machines is unpleasant. Maybe they're just imitating some hearing youngsters who have assured them that the island is bad.

Yes, I do have all these "children." My own boys are far away in our home country. Letters come in from Finland almost every week—mainly from Keke; Joppe doesn't write much.

The weekends are long for Jukka and me. We don't know what to do. Before, we always went to the Yacht Club and watched the boys sailing. But what would we do there now? We don't sail, nor do we enjoy sitting at the bar. Mary Charles has macrame as a hobby; she makes beautiful hanging flower baskets. Mary teaches me how to make knots, but macrame comes to a sudden end, because no string can be found on the island. Jukka goes to Spanish lessons, but then he doesn't have the time or the strength to continue.

We both are waiting for the end of May to arrive, when school will end and the boys will come to us for their vacation.

It's dry and sunny, and smaller and smaller streams of water come from the tap. I store refreshing moist towels in case there's a time when no water is available for washing up. Now water is saved, clothes are washed less often, the garden isn't watered, cars aren't washed.

Nature dries up more and more, and the sunlight changes to bright yellow when it doesn't sift through the thick green foliage. The leaves on the trees are dry, the grass is burned, the scenery looks more spacious. But there's not any extra humidity in the air, and it feels wonderful.

Anderson comes to work in the afternoons worn out and with his face all shining from sweat.

"Uh huh, it's very hot!"

It's very hot every day, and Anderson doesn't have the strength to work. He sits on the stairs in the shade, especially when nobody is at home. When Jukka comes home, nothing is done, and Jukka gets mad. I feel sorry for Anderson.

Anderson says that it's too hot to work and that he has a headache. But people say that it's only laziness. Anderson would much rather make beautiful flower arrangements for me than cut grass or clean the drains. He talks of all that he is going to do, and I'm grumpy because Jukka gives the orders to Anderson and I don't understand what Anderson is mumbling. I'm tired and cross about standing there trying to understand what Anderson is saying. That's what my life is like: I try to understand what other people are saying.

Finally the waiting comes to an end. Keke and Joppe have left Finland; they're in London now. (I wonder if they'll realize they must get their bags between planes, if they'll find the bus to the hotel; suppose they've forgotten to take their yellow vaccination cards with them?) Now they're on the plane on their way to St. Lucia, and Jukka calls the airline office and asks if the boys are on the plane. Then it's time for Jukka to go to the airport to meet them. Jeri and I wait on the balcony. I wonder if Jeri still knows the boys?

And finally, after it gets dark, the car drives up the hill. Jeri starts to bark; the car turns at our crossing and drives to the yard through the mango trees. Jeri barks and jumps up and down. Keke gets out of the car; he has become a man. And then Joppe, and Jukke carrying the suitcases. I have a lump in my throat. I have the boys back, but I feel oppressed already by another thought: this is only temporary, after a while we have to be apart again for months.

But now we celebrate the family's being together again, as we did before when Jukka came home from his ship. Back then, the boys and I were waiting, and I had the same kind of strangling feeling, that this is only temporary and we soon have to part. I'll be left in my miserable loneliness to look after the boys. I really don't know if it would be easier for me to be separated from the boys or from Jukka. There hasn't been much everyday routine in my life, only the pain of separation and then the time for celebration.

And gifts are always a part of the celebration, bagsful of all that you have longed for, so that suddenly you feel you're getting too much at one time. And the feeling of preparing evening tea for the whole family again, sitting with the entire family, and there's so much to talk about that you can't get started! It won't be till tomorrow that we read the boys' report cards—all their good grades . . . although it's not all that important that the grades are good.

Jeri gets his own dog bone and is chewing it on the mat. He won't understand until tomorrow that the boys have arrived, and I guess the same goes for me, too.

The boys inspect the house. They must sense the mixture of moisture and mosquito coils that hangs in the house. For them the sounds of the tropical night are strange; they have to get used to them all over again.

"It's good to be back. You just keep on staying here, so we can come here during our vacations."

The boys are pale after the dark Nordic winter. In the morning they wake up early and go out to play tennis and go swimming. Joppe covers his light skin with sun cream. In the evening the boys go to bed early, but soon their rhythm will change; they'll go to bed later and wake up later, and jet lag will subside. They'll no longer play tennis at five o'clock in the morning.

"I didn't remember that it's so warm here. We don't have the energy to do as much here as we do back home," Keke says.

I go shopping to buy food. I cook, bake, too little at first. It's mango time; Keke sits in the kitchen leaning over the sink, eating a juicy mango with juice all flowing down his chin. He's forgotten how to suck from under the peel as the locals do.

John Eugene is at our house constantly, as if he were our third son. He comes jogging to us along the beach in the morning coolness and leaves only after dinner. I feel that I'm living fully again, with all my old worries about the boys' well-being.

"Be careful, Joppe, that you don't burn. Come in out of the sun now. Cross the road carefully. Have some milk. Remember to put your lifejackets on when you go sailing . . ."

I'm incurable. Keke takes it all kindly, Joppe, irritably. But both of the boys emerge from the cotton I would like to wrap them in and climb the steep Petit Piton. They spend many hours on a walking tour in the jungle; they take a banana boat to Grenada, St. Vincent, Dominica. All I can do is pack clothes and a lunch and try not to worry about them.

In the evenings, Jukka and the boys play chess, or a conversation turns into an argument and Keke gets angry. So we're living a normal family life again.

Keke has a suit and tie with him, and I get the idea of sending him to a party in my place. Keke goes and represents me, and gets bored after two hours.

Our landlord Victor Archer is the deputy governor now, so on the Queen's Birthday I go to the reception again and stand on the lawn again in front of the Governor's House, with a glass in my hand.

DOING THE FOLLOW-UP

One Wednesday Joseph and Victor come, just the two of them, and tell me that Kenneth is "out," has been kicked out.

I don't quite understand what has happened, and Kenneth doesn't appear to tell me himself.

Joseph and Victor perform a pantomime of what has happened: Kenneth played instead of working, and Dave came over and spoke to him. Kenneth stood there defiantly, with his arms crossed over his chest, and Dave got mad and told him "Out!"

Jukka says that Kenneth is still too young and immature for work. When Kenneth doesn't appear for a long while, I ask Jukka to drive me by his house. I leave a message that "Raija hopes that Kenneth comes to Raija's home." I teach the sign to a woman who is Kenneth's "mother" at the moment. The house is new and clean, in the new Entrepot housing area.

And Kenneth does come, a bit defiant and sad, but there's not so much to worry about as I had imagined.

"Work?" he repeats.

Kenneth would like desperately to get work; he doesn't want just to be home. He wants to go to work, buy clothes, buy food, and take money home.

"Shoes bad. Give me shoes."

"Shirt bad. Give me shirt."

"I am hungry. I have not had lunch."

"Book?"

"We'll see. Maybe I'll find shoes somewhere that will fit. And we'll see, maybe we also can find work. But you're too young; you can't keep your job. Even now Dave told you 'Out!' What did you do?"

Kenneth's eyes burn; he gets excited as he performs pantomime of what happened. He is Dave and Kenneth in turn.

The scene is the dairy. Kenneth opens up canned-milk cans and sets them on the table. Dave comes, touches Kenneth's shoulder lightly; he wants to say something.

Later, Kenneth is still opening cans. Dave comes and pushes Kenneth's shoulder, Kenneth should open the cans faster and not think about anything else or look around.

Later, it's the same scene, but Dave comes and pokes Kenneth, irritated. Kenneth staggers a bit. He becomes defiant, turns away with his arms crossed, doesn't "listen" to what Dave has to say.

Dave lifts up his thumb and points to the door: Out.

So that's how it happened. Dave's behavior toward the deaf boys has changed gradually now that Clyde is no longer here to keep up positive attitudes. Dave hasn't always understood the deaf boys, he hasn't had enough means to express what he wanted to say. That's how he has become more and more irritated, especially when Kenneth has become more defiant the more difficult communication has become.

I explain to Kenneth that it's his fault. If his employer Dave says something, he has to obey, because Dave pays his salary. Kenneth gets his salary from doing what Dave tells him to do. He always has to smile politely and listen to what Dave wants to say, never being defiant.

"But Dave pushed."

"Yes, but in spite of that you still should have done what Dave told you, to open the cans as fast as possible, so that Joseph could have made more ice cream."

Again Kenneth shows how Dave pushed him, but I won't give in. Dave wouldn't have poked him if Kenneth's childish behavior hadn't irritated him. And now Kenneth has to stay at home long enough to become a little older and learn how to act at work. And while he's at home, he can learn more, more words, to count, to write. The more he learns, the easier it is for him to learn more.

I search for books for Kenneth. Count from that, read this. I'll see how many words you know.

I notice that Kenneth already knows how to count with single numbers; we can start with tens. Kenneth's vocabulary is bigger than I thought, because I didn't teach the fast group in school. Kenneth seems to know about a hundred English words. His passive vocabulary is even larger. Kenneth understands more words than he is able to spell. He really is gifted.

And Kenneth is studying eagerly; it's as if he's devouring knowledge. He appears on the balcony a couple of times a week. I don't say anything, I just bring juice and lemonade, because Kenneth has walked for three miles in the hot sunshine. Sometimes, when I'm having my afternoon nap, Joppe wakes me up and tells me that Kenneth is sitting on the balcony.

"OK, I'll come."

I don't ever say anything about books, but after finishing his juice, Kenneth says in his demanding style: "Books, pens."

I don't force Kenneth to learn; everything depends on him. But I don't need to force him. Kenneth has a strong will to learn.

Despite his eager studying, he doesn't forget to remind me every time about work.

"Write to Dave. I want to go back to work."

"No, Dave doesn't want to take you on."

Joseph is also sad. He too has difficulties at work, and they've threatened to put him out. A new bearded foreman doesn't like the boys at all and would like to get rid of them completely. He complains about them constantly to Dave.

I go to the dairy, talk to the manager with a paper and pen. He is polite. We have often met in passing at the Yacht Club.

No, Kenneth is too immature. Maybe sometime later . . .

I try to get Filipa to work at My Fair, but the matter comes down to her illiteracy. She needs to be able to read the instructions.

"Do you write the instructions also for the other deaf girls?" I ask the manager, surprised.

"Yes."

"And the girls understand?"

"Yes. Everything goes very well."

Is that so? I could tell him about those instructions. The girls have come to my house in the evenings after work and pulled papers out of their pockets, and I have interpreted them as best I can, usually without knowing the background. If I started to fight for Filipa to get work, the other girls' jobs would be endangered, and who would it all benefit then?

"I am sorry," the manager says.

So am I, truly, but you just say so because it's customary; it's a suitable way to wash your hands of the whole matter.

I go home and tell my story to Keke, who is sitting on the balcony reading. I sit opposite him, depressed. Keke makes cappuccino, brings me a cup and says that I don't need to care. But I do care for a long time. I'm bothered mostly because I haven't cared enough from the very beginning, as if I had given up before we started. As if I didn't have enough faith and only carried out my responsibilities according to the rules.

EXTENDED TIME

"**T**his is confidential information," Jukka says. "We made a plan for the use of the Cul-de-Sac's industrial area. An oil refinery will be built there. But other than the Prime Minister, nobody else knows about it yet."

An oil refinery! It's awful. It will spoil the whole island, destroy the whole idyll.

I don't understand. Jukka has made many good plans and carried through many fine projects, but now I don't understand why he is in the group that wants to spoil one of the few unspoiled places left on earth, where the water and air are still clean.

"It doesn't have to spoil anything, if it is well taken care of. People need work and bread."

I know that, but how often there have been two opposing sides: on one, the pollution of the air and water and the spoiling of nature, and on the other, people's livelihood. I know what kind of poverty the idyll of this island hides. It's not the biggest misery in the world, but can you compare miseries?

I think of children who run around in the villages of the banana plantations with swollen bellies, of old men who sleep on cardboard on the loading docks of the storehouses near the port, of about two hundred boys and eighty girls who live under boats and beg in the streets. I think of the ever-growing population of youth, like a time bomb, unemployed. The politicians know it; that's why they so eagerly want some industry on the island.

Jukka has contacted many Finnish firms. Maybe one of them could set up a factory here. Some Finns are interested already and intend to visit St. Lucia.

In any case, I'm happy that I got to live on the island during the time when it was still untouched and unspoiled.

Jukka has done his work well; he is offered extended time. The port has become profitable. It pays for itself, and there's even money saved for other expenses of the island state. The Castries Port is becoming the training center for the small states in the Caribbean. The training is paid by the Caribbean Development Bank. Jukka guides and looks after all this.

I don't have anything against spending still another year on the island. I'm getting comfortable with my life over here; the circles have become familiar. An extra year will deepen the circles, although I think that three years is enough. There will be nothing new for us any more by then.

People come and go, experts and volunteers come, stay a while, leave. You always have to keep saying farewell. I keep hoping there will be someone among the newcomers whom I can make friends with. Finally I stop hoping; I get used to the fact that I have some acquaintances, but no real friends. Friends are in my home country and the mail moves between us. Kaisu writes letters ten pages long. I answer. Jukka listens to music, says it relaxes him. I don't say anything, but I feel a sting. I would like to listen to music myself. I remember what it's like. But I write letters. I tell everything I have inside of me. To Kaisu and Ella, Rea and Aura.

Yes, I can take another year over here. An economic depression awaits me in Finland; it's easy for me over here, but I fear that I'm getting lazy. I don't have as much energy to move around and hustle as I do back home.

The boys leave for Finland. I won't see them again until after the term is over in the spring.

I'm sitting on the balcony again, watching the sunset; rats are running along the telephone lines and down the poles, geckos appear at their catching stations on the balcony, bats flap around looking for holes in the ceiling.

I would like to do so much over here, but there's not much I can do. I've tried, but I couldn't help, or I've helped in the wrong way. And how much this wet heat tires you! I don't get used to it—on the contrary, I've given in to it. I don't feel guilty any more that I sleep a lot. In the evenings my feet are like bundles of lead, and my limbs are weary, even when I haven't done anything at all.

There are new hearing teachers at the school. For them I am something less than what I was for Clyde—I am disabled. I'm not needed at the school. Millie sees me in a different light, but for her the deaf world is as close as it is for me. Millie opens up new possibilities for me by interpreting the society's meetings for me in sign language.

Sometimes on Sundays when we drive up to the mountains I see people who sit doing nothing on the porches of their small houses. They look as if they've been sitting there for a long time, without any hurry, in the Sunday peace. Sometimes they watch what's going on around them, sometimes they don't see anything. Maybe they aren't even thinking of anything.

I often sit on the balcony myself—just sit and think. I feel the wind around me, or raindrops, or the sun, whose rays fill every place so that even in the shade I can feel my skin becoming weather-beaten and smell it as it tans.

And in my thoughts I watch the scenery that has become so familiar to me: blue bay, lighthouse on the other side. The round palm tops that frame it, the red ceiling against the blue sky. Or I look at my friends, the green lizards that catch insects in the afternoon warmth.

I notice how good it is, sometimes, to sit without doing anything, let the thoughts wander, become bright and pop into an idea—a beginning for something new. I wonder where the notion has come from that a human being has to hustle all the time, to keep going like a machine, to feel guilty if she sits down even for a moment.

Zenia has another baby. Zenia's world lies between her home and our house, a small room in the mountains and her children. She nevers goes to the beach or outside of the town farther than our house. I would like to tell her that it is possible for her to have another fifteen babies, how could she manage with such a mob of children? But what good would it do for me to say anything; it's none of my business. Maybe, at bottom, I'm just envious of her unshaken peace of mind.

Jukka has got us a new maid. Lucy is here by seven, preparing breakfast. When we eat, Lucy brings a tray with a piece of bread on it—for Jeri. Jeri is like a prince to her. Mornings he sleeps on the bed, with his head on the pillow. During the night it's impossible for him to sleep, for he has to listen to every sound of the tropical night, and early in the morning he has to bark at all the passersby going to work and to school. In the afternoons he's on guard as Lucy carefully mixes his food: crushed biscuits in cooked rice.

Lucy does everything—she even brings me my morning coffee on a tray at ten o'clock. If I do anything, she feels offended. I make my own bed, no matter how fine a lady I otherwise am. I don't know what kind of role Lucy expects me to play; I imagine it originated with her former lady.

Okay, I am like ladies in English novels. In the mornings I take care of correspondence, make out shopping lists, write instructions for Lucy about our meals. Handiwork and reading . . . I keep my shoes on at all times. And I put on a necklace and dab perfume behind my ears. Maybe I'll get tired of playing the role of a fine lady, tomorrow or the day after, surely next week. I don't enjoy roles very long, either the ones I'm pressed into or the ones I adopt once in a while— cleaning fanatic or the dedicated housewife who cooks and bakes and keeps the place tip-top. But let's see how long this lasts without our fighting.

I take a day at a time as it comes and see what happens.

John Eugene arrives, bringing his report card. John is looking for a job and is worried because jobs aren't easy to find. I give him lunch and dinner; he can have an old pair of Keke's pants and a shirt Keke doesn't wear any more. John is satisfied; he looks well-dressed and presentable. But usually he just sits on the balcony for days, staring straight ahead or dozing; sometimes his eyes are sad and empty. He comes so often that I become tired of it, but how can I tell a depressed and hungry boy that he can't come and see me?

Joseph, Kenneth, and Victor come as well. I bring food to the table, ask for their news. Kenneth has found a job at the supermarket; he is happy and signs with liveliness. The new black-bearded boss at the creamery has finally fired Victor.

"Work?" Victor signs many times, opening his hands questioningly.

"I think, I try." I am not sure if I will be able to look for a job for Victor. I don't seem to have the strength for it.

I give the boys bus fare so that they don't need to walk. Darkness falls quite suddenly.

"Wednesday?"

"Yes, do come on Wednesday again."

Magilda doesn't come on Wednesday. She comes on Saturday, saying that she has a headache and that's why she left work early.

Magilda is worried; Valerie is expecting a baby. Magilda doesn't have any intention of having a baby; she wants to work. Now Magilda is sick, but not because she is expecting a baby.

Magilda is having breakfast with us. She asks to see the photo albums that she has looked through dozens of times, but which still always interest her.

"How about if Magilda would start expecting a baby anyhow? You never know."

Magilda has doubts. Maybe the fear has been in her mind from the beginning; maybe that's why she has come to me.

"All girls—school finish—then baby."

Magilda has at least ten rings, one on almost all her fingers, two on some of them.

"Boyfriend give."

"You have a boyfriend?"

Magilda nods.

"Baby comes very easily. If you sleep with your boyfriend, baby can come. One or two times . . . If you only walk or kiss, no baby."

How can I explain it any better? How can I explain this to a deaf girl so that it will fit into her mind-set? How much sex education can you give in this culture? I don't know. I only hope that whatever I say will help Magilda, at least for a while.

"Baby. Work out," Magilda says. "Salary good. Four violet, two green, and one red note. Last week there were only two violet notes, and all women were angry and threw the money in their purses."

The following Wednesday the boys also know about Valerie.

"Stupid," Kenneth signs.

But Valerie is said not to mind at all; she is satisfied. She has always wanted a baby, and now she will get one. She's too simple to worry about anything. Not even that almost all her teeth are already broken or gone.

Because I mentioned it, Theresa is now unhappy because of the big black holes in her front teeth. But now that she has finally gone to the dental clinic, it turns out to be too late. The holes can't be filled any more. Later, when the holes are very big, the teeth will be pulled, and Theresa is unhappy. If I hadn't said anything, Theresa would consider the matter irrelevant, and wouldn't care. The teeth are simply "finished." It happens a lot.

The boys are also interested in girls. Victor and Kenneth have started to go to the Baptist Church. Now they go to lessons every evening. In the church there are girls who are interested in them. Victor giggles and Kenneth and Victor get fits when they think of the girls in the church, and all Joseph can do is watch quietly. Not until Jukka comes home is Victor quiet, and even Joseph gets his turn.

Jukka makes the boys water the garden, and Victor invents a name sign for Jukka: "Captain Who Commands."

I wonder about Kenneth. He's found himself a job, and he goes to church now. And although he doesn't understand everything, he understands quite a lot. The boys have to communicate with the people around them at least somewhat, and I want to know how it happens. How do deaf people become even this well integrated with hearing people, considering that most people know hardly anything about deafness, and their attitudes are sometimes strange? Is it that Kenneth, Victor, and Joseph have strong self-confidence, and when they respect themselves, others also respect them? The fact that Kenneth can even work in the store is a wonder, because hearing is especially important in a store.

I go to town, I'm walking, deep in my thoughts, along the hot boulevard. Somebody tugs at my sleeve, stands in front of me. I look up, narrowing my eyes. Alfonso is standing in front of me: beautiful, grown-up, his hair curly under the cap that the rastafarians wear. He greets me, friendly and smiling, as if he's forgotten all grudges.

"You well?"

Alfonso points to the ice cream carriage further down the Boulevard in front of the cinema.

"You sell ice cream?"

Alfonso nods.

"You get money?"

Again Alfonso nods.

"You buy food. Where home?"

Alfonso points to the mountains.

"Rain. Cold. I to your house."

I tell him that I'll think about it. I don't know why I always promise, because I know already that we can't take him in again. I could give him money, but not my own time and strength. It's easy to give money, but to give something from oneself—that is more difficult.

I wouldn't have the strength to get involved so deeply in John Eugene's concerns, but he comes in the mornings, sits on the balcony all day, comes with me to the beach. He stands as if rooted next to the almond tree. The hotel guard comes to send him away, but John doesn't leave. He says that he's with me. The sand and water are for everyone, nobody can be driven away from the beach, and yet John stands on the grass under the almond tree instead, as if in protest.

The local boys on the beach are boisterous and noisy and yell impudent comments at the tourists. Millie says I can feel lucky that I don't hear what they yell at the white people.

I no longer dare to go anywhere but to the hotel beach, because the island belongs to the local inhabitants; the water and the sand are theirs. What do they care if the tourists won't come a second time because of their impoliteness? Who cares if the noise disturbs the tourists' sleep on their beach chairs under the palms? In the funny clothes they wear, even to town, tourists are objects of contempt, and so are all white people on the island.

I get my share of the local people's spite. When I go to the supermarket, the boys who pack the bags and cart them to the car are unwilling and impolite. If we complain to their bosses, it doesn't help any, because they're on the boys' side. Mostly whites shop at the supermarket, because it carries the imported goods that the locals don't buy. The whites cart away expensive food every week, their shopping baskets overflowing. Every time I pay the cashier I'm aware that the total for that day's shopping is the same as Lucy and others get paid in a month. But nothing can be done about it. I change stores; that much I can do. I start going to the J. Q. Charles Supermarket in town, where there's a sense of the island's spirit. I buy the same goods the locals do.

One morning John Eugene is happy—finally he can get a job at a hotel. He must take his medical records and identity card to his employer. But his black shoes won't do, and neither will his shirt. John doesn't have money to buy new ones. Because he doesn't have work, he doesn't have money, and because he doesn't have money, he can't go to work. Without papers, good black shoes, and a new white shirt, John can't get started.

But John does have us. I write a check and promise to talk to Jukka about the shoes. Maybe we'll even buy the shirt. John takes the check casually, without thanks. I tell him that the money is a loan, and when John has money, he has to take care of himself. John doesn't thank us now, but at Christmas and on Mother's Day he brings a card in which he thanks us with beautiful words. I just have to remember those cards when John, looking proud, with his head upright and saying nothing, takes the money, food, pants, socks, everything that we give him.

I learn that Alfonso's behavior wasn't so strange after all. He is more an islander than a deaf person. He did as it is the way on the island to do, and we expected him to behave according to our customs.

And why, after all, should these boys be grateful to me? I give to them because I have some source to give from, while they on their part hardly have anything. It's I who should be thankful for what I have and for the fact that, once in a while, I can experience the joy of giving. If I could, I would give from what I have so that we all could have the same amount.

But I can always take a brown paper bag from the cupboard, fill it up, and take lunch to school for those children who don't have any lunch with them. I can take eggs and ask that they be boiled for them. Gradually others get interested; we cook more and more so that all deaf children finally get lunch at school.

I can fill up the bag for Zenia, Anderson, John. It will help them through at least one day. The supply of food never seems to run out. There seems to be more money for helping than for my own unnecessary expenses. Money is not what it looks like; it's all relative. And even helping is a relative matter, as you can't always know what effect you've had and when you've helped most. You never know if you would have helped more in some way that you didn't even notice. That's how it should be: the left hand doesn't know what the right hand is doing.

Sometimes we drive to the beach of the Cariblue Hotel. There I look at people who sail in their boats, bask on the beach, ride motorboats, and sweep past on water skis. They have money, and they're well fed, and they're having a good time, but they are here escaping their own worries and sorrows for a while.

In their nonchalance these vacationers arouse hatred in people who live on the island and see a glimpse of a world where everything looks easy. They see that others have more money than they. And sometimes some tourist is acting difficult. In any of the hotels there are always guests who show off and start trouble as if to show that it's they who are paying here. The boys who serve them think that's what all white people are like. I don't make this up myself; John has told me about it.

As we sit on the balcony in the evenings, I gradually begin to feel as if we're cutting loose from everything. There's a cocktail party going on somewhere right this moment. We have fallen out of this whole well-woven network. Of course, it's due somewhat to my deafness, but it's not solely because of that. If we had decided to take our places in the network, we could have done it in one way or another.

The fact that I have a hearing impairment doesn't mean the same thing as before. Deafness is a part of me, part of my life. Without it I wouldn't be what I am, and I wouldn't have done what I've done. I can't deny it and say that deafness is nothing, that there are no problems, that I don't care at all whether I can hear or not. I do care sometimes; I care a whole lot, so much that it hurts.

However, I can see problems all around me that are so much worse—on the island, in my home country, everywhere—and in the small circles of island people the problems seem to take over. Jealousy, poverty, grudges, greediness, hatred, violence . . . and I'm sure that any one of those emotions makes the person whom it possesses more miserable than deafness has made me.

We have to think of returning to our own country. But not yet—we're living in St. Lucia time; the voyage to the island has not yet ended. And I know that the island will follow me back to my home country, as an experience that changed me, causing me to see everything differently. That's why my voyage to the island will never end. 🍁

EPILOGUE

F rom the beginning of the twentieth century until the seventies, many countries prohibited the use of sign language in the education of the deaf, and Finland was no exception. Its deaf people had no right to use their own language. In 1970, however, the status of sign language gradually began to improve. The Finnish Association of the Deaf (FAD) published a *Pictorial Dictionary of Sign Language*, and some hearing people became interested in this language and wanted to learn it.

I left Finland for St. Lucia in 1975; I went armed with a certificate testifying that I was qualified to teach sign language. At that time, the FAD's small office in Helsinki served 2,500 members—out of the 5,000 deaf people in Finland (8,000 if we include those deafened)—with only a director and one full-time assistant.

When I returned to Finland in 1979 I realized that I had learned, used, and taught Signed Finnish, not Finnish Sign Language (FSL). Signed Finnish was no longer being taught, and FSL was in use all over the country. In St. Lucia I had seen how important sign language is for deaf children; now I saw how important it is for all deaf Finns to have the right to use FSL.

The FAD office had moved to larger quarters, where seven persons now worked. Liisa Kauppinen was then FAD director. I started working for the FAD immediately after my return, first as a secretary, but with responsibility also for FAD cultural activities. From 1982 to 1985 I served as secretary for the committee on Deaf Culture, set up by the Finnish Ministry of Education. We prepared a comprehensive report not only on the performing arts, but on the entire situation of deaf people in Finland.

In 1984 I became cultural officer of the FAD, and in January 1987, director of the Cultural Centre. Today, in our very large, new offices in the Centre Malminharju and in local offices all over the country, the FAD now employs ninety-five people. The association is a federation of fifty-two local deaf clubs; it provides various sign language services, and looks after the interests of the deaf community.

The deaf community in Finland is more visible now than ever before, mainly because FSL has been accepted. Deaf people have many technical devices to make their everyday life easier. Video programs produced by Deaf Video furnish information in sign language. Interpreter services are available for all, including deaf students in different schools, colleges, and universities. More parents of deaf children learn to sign. During my first working days in 1979, I learned a new term: deaf awareness. Nowadays we can proudly live as deaf persons in Finland.

Facing the problems and prejudices still to be overcome, including raising the status of FSL in deaf education, my personal goal as FAD cultural director is to help give deaf people opportunities to produce cultural services. We want to strengthen the cultural identity of deaf adults and support deaf children and their families so that children will discover their cultural identity.

We are now living in Helsinki, three miles from my office. My husband Jukka is working as a private management consultant, mainly in international port-related projects financed by the Finnish International Development Agency, the African Development Bank, the Asian Development Bank, and the World Bank. During the last five years, these projects have concentrated on East Africa and Southeast Alsia.

Keijo (Keke) is a medical doctor. Jorma (Joppe) is studying at Helsinki University of Technology and working with IBM. Our dog Jeri died one year after flying back from St. Lucia. Rottweiler Tito has replaced him as an important family member.

In 1982 Jukka and I visited St. Lucia and saw all our dear friends there. Then in 1989, we attended the Deaf Way Congress in Washington, D.C., we took advantage of the opportunity and continued our trip to St. Lucia. I visited the school for the deaf and all the places where my former pupils were working. Kenneth, who has written to me regularly and sent me newspapers and clippings, is working in an educational equipment store. Joseph and Victor are still working at Ferrand's Dairy, while Theresa is working at My Fair. Valerie has at least two babies. The younger pupils, who were in the infant class, are now grown up and have jobs. Everyone I saw was neatly dressed and well behaved; it was a pleasure to see my former pupils doing so well. I asked them if they saw each other after work, and they answered, "We are always together." They clearly have formed the deaf community on the island although they do not yet have any formal organization of the deaf.

I did not go to see Alfonso. It would have been too difficult for both of us. In 1985 Kenneth had sent me a clipping of the *Voice*, describing five homes built by the St. Lucia government for homeless people. In one of the pictures was Alfonso, smiling—but sightless. Having lost his vision, Alfonso is now both deaf and blind.

I have not heard from Clyde Vincent, with whom I worked so hard teaching deaf children. However, I have kept in contact with his successor, Millie Brother. To my great pleasure, Millie stayed at our home for one week during the World Congress of the World Federation of the Deaf in 1987. We share a love for St. Lucia School for the Deaf, and both are happy that the school has made such good progress. The school has recently been given a plot of land for a new schoolhouse. Mrs. Cynthia Weekes told me about her dream to build a dormitory so that all the deaf children on the island could come to school. Relatively little money is needed for the dormitory, but it is difficult to raise the funds. I hope that by my next visit to the island, her dream has become a reality.